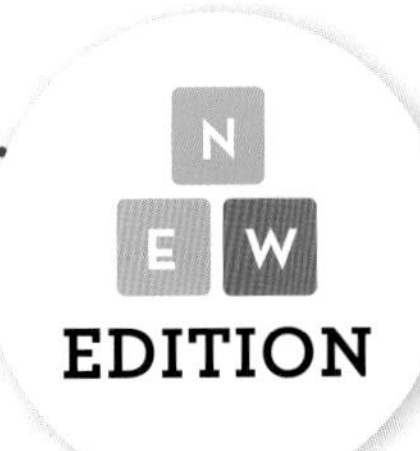

25 Things Every New Mom Should Know

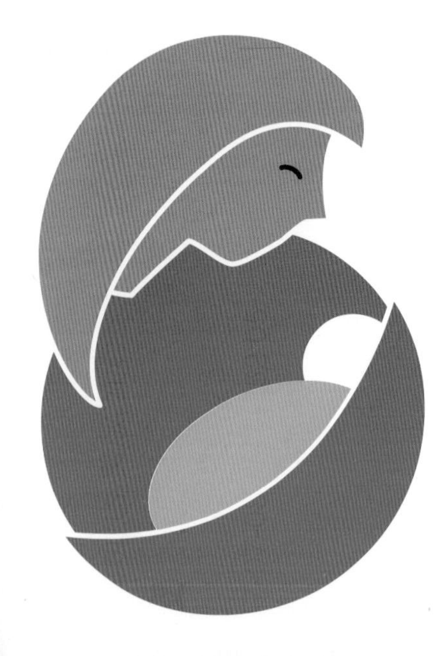

MARTHA SEARS, R.N., WITH **WILLIAM SEARS, M.D.**
THE AUTHORS OF *THE BABY BOOK*

NEW EDITION

25 Things Every New Mom Should Know

Essential First Steps for Mothers

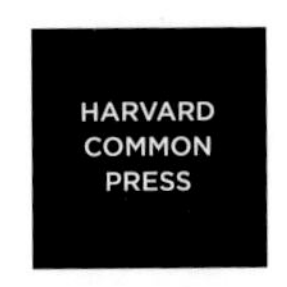

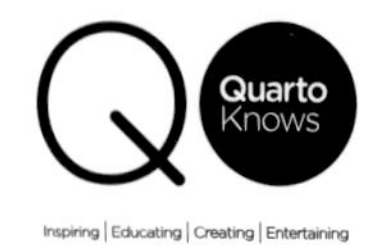

First Published in 2017 by The Harvard Common Press, an imprint of The Quarto Group,
100 Cummings Center, Suite 265-D, Beverly, MA 01915, USA.
T (978) 282-9590 F (978) 283-2742 QuartoKnows.com

The Harvard Common Press titles are also available at discount for retail, wholesale, promotional, and bulk purchase. For details, contact the Special Sales Manager by email at specialsales@quarto.com or by mail at The Quarto Group, Attn: Special Sales Manager, 401 Second Avenue North, Suite 310, Minneapolis, MN 55401, USA.

21 20 19 18 17 1 2 3 4 5

ISBN: 978-1-55832-892-1

Digital edition published in 2017

Originally found under the following Library of Congress Cataloging-in-Publication Data
Sears, Martha.
25 things every new mother should know / by Martha Sears, with William Sears.
p. cm.
Includes bibliographical references.
ISBN 1-55832-068-7 — ISBN 1-55832-069-5 (pbk.)
1. Infants (Newborn)—Care. 2. Infants—Care. 3. Mother and infant. I. Sears, William, M.D.
II. Title. III. Title: Twenty-five things every new mother should know.
RJ253.S397 1995
659'.122—dc20 94-47976

Printed in China

Acknowledgment

We would like to thank

Gwen Gotsch

for her contribution to this book.

Contents

Introduction ... 9

1 Giving Birth Is a Complex Emotional Experience ... 15

2 A Newborn Baby Is Already a Person ... 23

3 You and Your Baby Need to Stay Together ... 31

4 Breastfeeding Really Is Better Than Bottle-Feeding ... 39

5 You Can Solve Breastfeeding Problems ... 47

6 New Mothers Need Special Care ... 55

7 All Your Energy Goes to the Baby ... 61

8 Your Baby Needs Your Help When She Cries ... 69

9 Your Baby Needs You Close by Day ... 77

10 Your Baby Needs You Close by Night ... 85

11 Beware the Self-Soothing Baby ... 95

12 You Really Do Have Intuition ... 101

13 Things Will Never Be "Normal" Again ... 107

14 Playtime Is All the Time ... 111

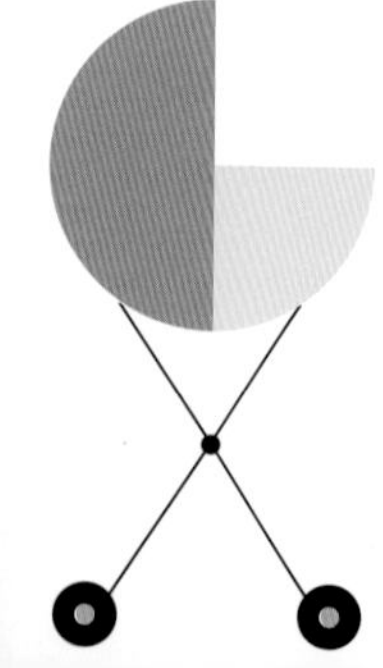

15 You Can Get the Baby's Father Involved 121

16 It's All Right to Feel Like Crying.............................. 129

17 Fathers Go On Being Husbands; Parents Are Still Lovers 137

18 Staying Home With Your Baby Can be
Practical and Rewarding 145

19 If You Go Back to Work, You'll Still be the Person Most
Important to Your Baby 151

20 Some Babies Are More Challenging Than Others 159

21 Continuing to Breastfeed Is Worth the Effort 165

22 You Are the Expert On Your Baby 173

23 You Need People to Lean On 181

24 You Don't Have to be Perfect 187

25 How You Mother Your Baby Does Make a Difference 195

Resources 201

The "Caveman" Diet 206

About the Authors 207

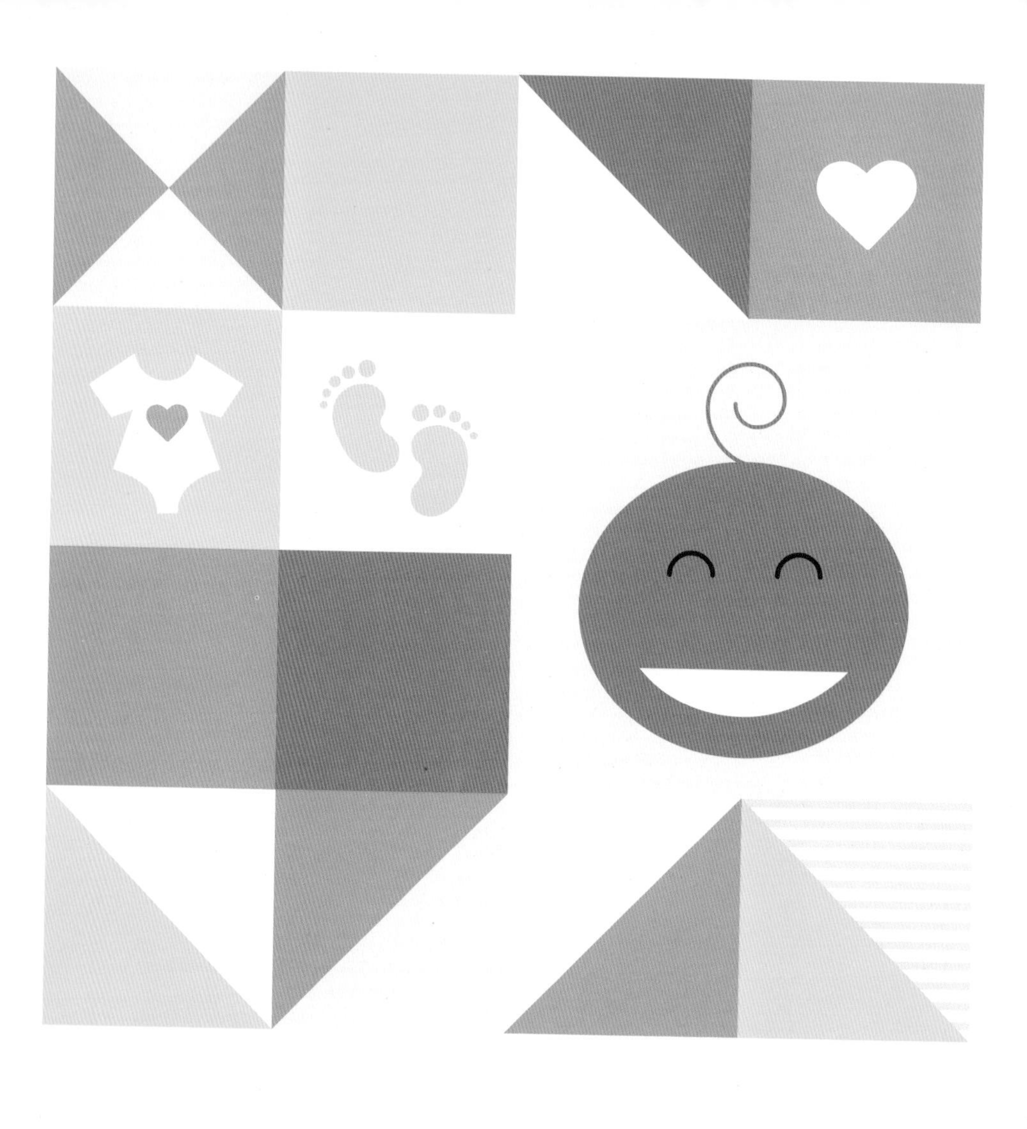

Introduction

Over 50 years ago I (Martha) became a mother for the first time. Even though I had "R.N." after my name I was pretty frightened. All those babies I'd played "Mommy" with in the hospital were other people's babies, not my own. I had to learn how to be a mother to my little Jimmy from scratch. It was intense and personal learning, and I have been privileged to experience it intensely and personally seven more times.

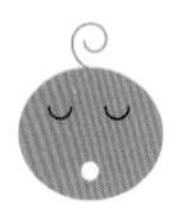

"We believe that babies have a lot to teach mothers."

My husband, Bill, learned along with me all the things we discuss in this book for brand-new mothers. My voice, speaking mother-to-mother, will dominate the book, with Bill's interjected here and there to give his perspective as a father and pediatrician.

This is not a traditional baby-care book. You won't find anything in it about diaper rash, cord care, or how to give a bath. You can get that information from a lot of other sources. Instead, this book is a guide to mothering your baby, and it is as much about the process of becoming a mother as it is about babies. It will help you to get to know your baby better, and we hope that it will also help you understand yourself as you take on this new, motherly role.

We believe that babies have a lot to teach mothers. Listening to your baby and responding to his or her cues will lead you into a parenting style that will help both of you thrive. Biology and infant behavior will help you get started and build your confidence as you and your baby develop a two-way trusting relationship. But this is not an ideal world we live in, and there are forces you'll meet along the way that can make you doubt your mothering intuition. We hope that this book will prepare you for some of those bumps in the road and will help you meet the challenges and changes ahead.

Mothering and fathering eight children has taught us a lot. We are very different persons from the ones we were before we had children, and most, if not all, of these differences are for the better. Although personal growth is sometimes hard, we've had a lot of fun along the way. Fun in your life with your baby is what will convince you and the baby that life is good.

Enjoy your baby!

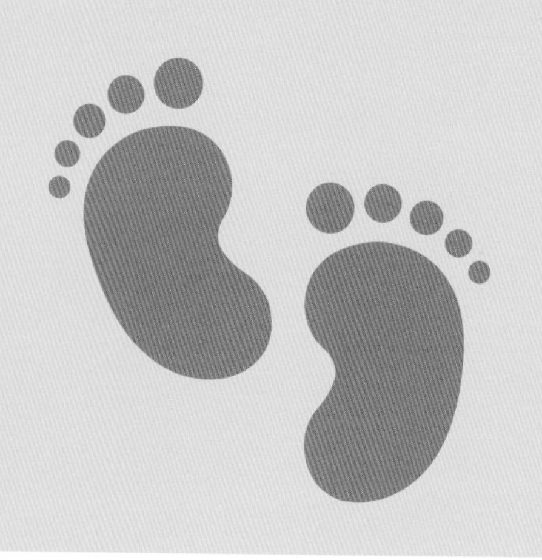

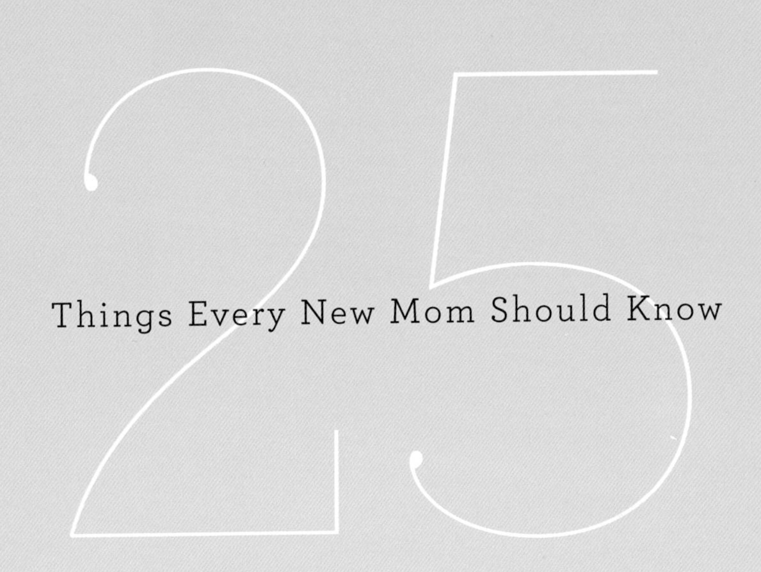

25 Things Every New Mom Should Know

MAMA
1

Giving Birth Is a Complex Emotional Experience

Suddenly—finally—you're not pregnant anymore! Gone is the great big bulge—the bumps that were knees and elbows, the big round head your health-care provider located at each prenatal checkup, the bulk that made it hard to breathe, hard to sleep, hard to roll out of bed in the morning. The heartbeat you've been listening to for over six months; the little thumps; the long, rib-tickling sweeps across your abdomen; the powerful jabs that made you wonder what you had in there—all of this and more is gone from inside you.

No more worrying about the birth. No more heartburn, or backache. No more watching your stomach jump while you sit perfectly still. No more preoccupation with the awesome fact of your own private miracle. Pregnancy's over, and it's time to meet your baby.

So how do you feel at this enormous moment in your life, the beginning of your mothering career? Sweaty? Chilled? Totally in awe, shaken, and shaking? Covered with bloody birth stuff? Relieved that the contractions have ended? Numb (literally or figuratively) from the chest down? Elated? Confused? All of these?

Nothing I say could ever completely prepare you for that moment when you first say hello to your baby. Every mother is different, every birth is different. But one thing I can tell you: Having a baby is a powerful event. It doesn't matter whether your labor was short or long, whether the birth was vaginal or cesarean, who is with you, or where you are. The emotions are big, as befits a time of great and sudden change.

I hope that for you those first moments of being a mother include seeing and touching and holding your baby. A new baby fresh from the warm, wet womb belongs in the mother's arms—a new sort of womb, and home for the next several months. So, too, do you, the new mother, need to physically experience the slippery little person with the squished-up face who moments before was still inside you. "Oh, baby! My baby," exalts the new mother. Seeing, touching, smelling, examining make the baby real to you. It is your way of knowing that your baby is alive, and yours.

This is your first job as a new mother—taking the psychological and emotional leap from pregnancy into parenthood. For nine months you carried this life hidden within your body, as someone both familiar and strange. Now the baby is here in the world for all to see, and your relationship with him is no longer so exclusive. The doctor examines him. Your partner gets to hold him. Nurses weigh him and check his temperature. Your baby has already started down the road to independence from you, though he does not know it; and you may feel that he is very much still a part of you. He moves his arm a certain way and you think, "Yes, I recognize that motion. You did that inside of me. I know you." Then, you gaze into his face and wonder, "Who are you, baby? Tell me who you are."

Give yourself the time and space to feel all these things. In all the hustle and bustle that surrounds birth, it's easy to be distracted or overwhelmed. Now is the time to be absorbed in your baby. Hold him next to your skin, let him gaze into your eyes, help him to find your nipple, give him the comfort and security of your arms after his incredible journey. Tell your birth team what you need; ask them to show you how to hold your baby so

Don't panic if the earth doesn't move for you in your first moments of motherhood.

he can rest, peaceful and quiet. If medical conditions prevent you from being able to hold your baby, insist that you at least see him and touch him, nuzzle him up close and smell him. If you can't be with your baby, plan for your partner to stay with him, talking and touching, so he's with one of his parents and can be comforted by someone he knows.

You may feel a wave of instant and overpowering love for your baby. You may feel wonder or awe. You might feel like laughing or crying tears of relief. Or you may feel just plain exhausted. All of these feelings are normal. Accept them. Don't panic if the earth doesn't move for you in your first moments of motherhood. There's a lot going on inside you, and it's going to take a few days to sort it all out.

Much discussion has gone on about "birth bonding," the idea that being with your baby in the hour or so after birth is critical to the formation of the parent-child relationship. Here's the truth about this "bonding" period. Yes, bonding with the baby is critical. However, being together in the first hour after birth is not a kind of magic glue that cements the parent-child relationship for all time. Bonding with your baby will be an ongoing process. The two of you will bond even if you do miss out on this first opportunity, whether for solid medical reasons or because of inane hospital routines.

Even so, early and intimate contact with your baby is important, because it helps you feel like your baby's mother that much sooner, and how you feel as a mother matters. It matters to you, and it matters to your baby. Your need to be with your baby is not touchy-feely nonsense. It is part of your intuitive drive to do the very best you can for your child. This need deserves respect and accommodation.

Your birth experience should be respected also—by you as well as by the people around you. Childbirth seldom turns out exactly as expected. As a woman who has given birth seven times (our eighth child is ours by adoption), I can tell you that no two of those experiences were the same. In the days to come, as you think back on the birth of your baby, you may wish you had done some things differently. For example, you may be unhappy, even heartsick, about having had a cesarean. You may not like the way someone treated you. Accept these feelings, but also recognize them as the inevitable product of hindsight. Don't fault yourself for your actions during labor. No one thinks clearly when contractions are coming every two minutes, with no time in between to rest, let alone collect your thoughts. The decisions you made during labor (even those made for you) were made with the best interests of your baby and yourself in mind. Even if you now perceive the situation differently than you did then, use this as an opportunity to learn and grow (and perhaps prepare for next time), rather than to beat up on yourself. Your baby's mother deserves better.

Digesting your birth experience is an important part of becoming a mother. You need to ponder. You need to tell your story over and over. How long was your labor? How did it feel? What did your caregivers say? Exactly what happened? Wise, experienced nurses, midwives, and doctors know that getting it all straight in your mind helps you incorporate your birth story into your life story. Other women who've had babies know this as well. So tell your story. Tell it with your partner, tell it to your friends, share it with your mother, *before* you look at photos or watch the video tape (you want to be able to always see this birth from within you). If something happened that you don't understand, ask someone who was there—your partner, a nurse, your doctor or midwife—to explain it to you or help you recall the event. This birth experience is a part of you now, and many years hence you'll still be able to describe it in great detail. When you have time (do it soon because newly born babies sleep a lot in the first few days), write your story down. Write a poem! If you are not creative, who is?

Entering motherhood is like any other transition in life in that it entails both a gain and a loss. I don't have to tell you that what you've gained is a whole new person to love, who will love you back. The loss is not quite so obvious. Leaving pregnancy behind is not always easy. When you were pregnant, you felt special. People took care of you. You babied yourself. Your partner fussed over you, carried the groceries, brought you treats. After the birth, the spotlight shifts to the baby, and you're the one doing the caregiving. Finding it hard to make this shift doesn't mean you're unhappy about or jealous of the baby. It does mean you still need someone to care for *you*, which I'll talk more about later.

Ceasing to be pregnant also means that you can leave the emotional issues of pregnancy behind. The reality of minute-to-minute baby care will soon turn you into an experienced mom. I hope that during your pregnancy you had a chance to think about the changes motherhood will bring, both to you as an individual and to your life with your partner. Talking about this during pregnancy can make the first months of parenthood easier. If there are problems left over from your nine months of gestating, recognize them when they pop up again in the weeks to come. Now that your baby is here, you will need to deal with them wisely and with kid gloves.

Suddenly—finally—you're not pregnant anymore. Get ready to meet your baby!

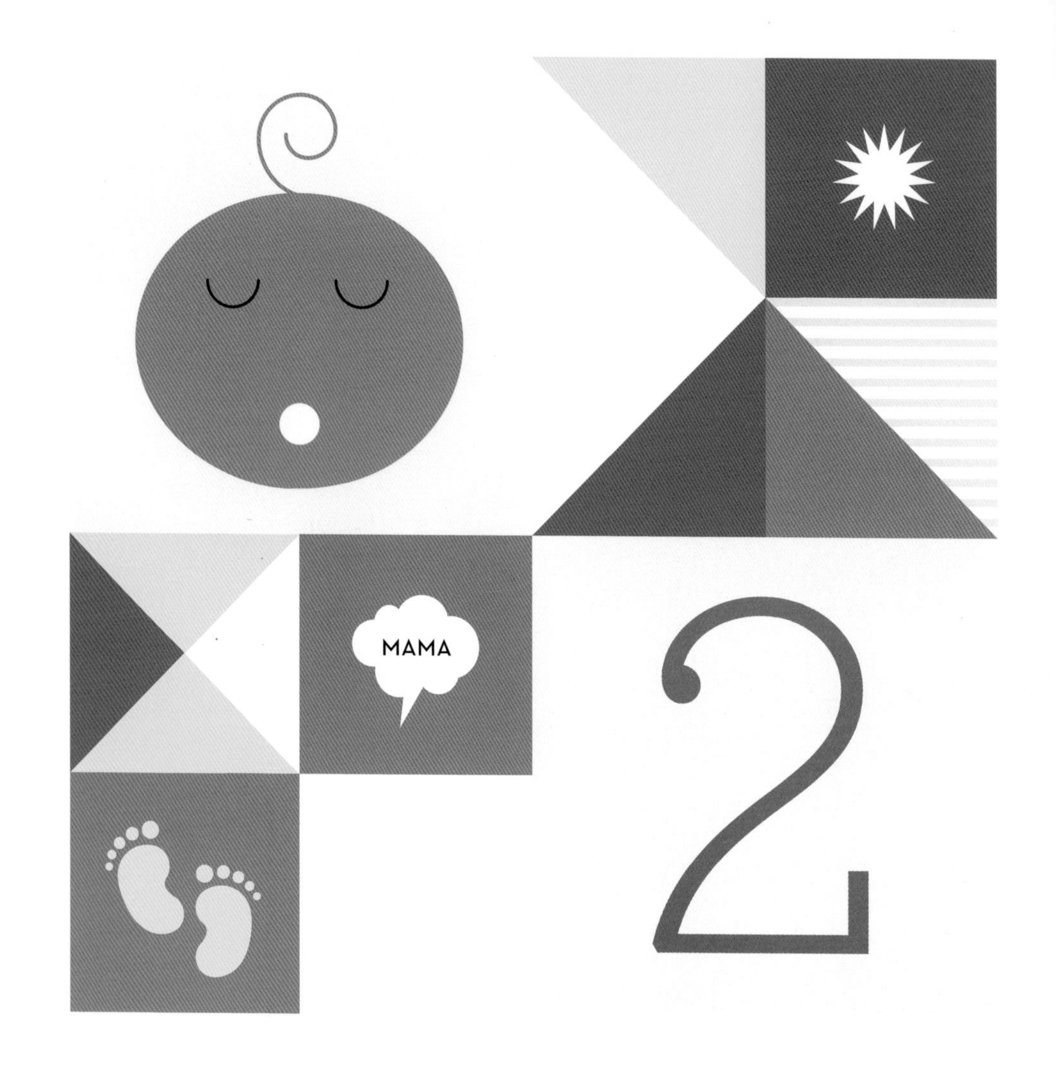
MAMA
2

A Newborn Baby Is Already a Person

A baby is a unique individual, right from the start. She is herself, a special human being with a personality all her own and a surprising number of well-developed abilities. Approach her with the same respect you would offer a fully grown human being. You and your baby are nine months into the great adventure the two of you will share; continue your journey by getting to know one another.

How do you handle a brand-new baby? You may feel awkward at first. Her head is floppy, though even now you may see your little one try to hold her head or at least turn it right again when it gets away from her. Every baby is different: Some love to be cuddled upright on Mom's chest or against her shoulder. Some want to be cradled in Mom's arms, even when they're not feeding. If it seems to you that your baby has a definite preference, you're probably right—and you've learned something about this little person.

I don't have to tell you to move gently and slowly with your newborn. You'll probably do this intuitively. Remember that up until now this baby has been floating in water, which cushioned her against your stopping, starting, and stepping. Sudden motions can make newborns startle; they throw their arms out to the sides and jerk their heads. They have an inborn fear of falling; if you had fur, your baby would cling to you, just like the baby apes who ride their mothers' backs at the zoo. If you are feeling stiff and achy from the birth, careful movements will feel best to you, too.

Try to find a position that allows your baby to feel comfortable and you to gaze right into her face. Support her head with one hand and her bottom with the other, and hold her directly in front of you. Make a baby-seat of your legs by bending them up on the bed in front of you, and lean your baby against your legs, facing you. Or lie down next to her, side by side, with her face even with yours. Take the time to really observe her, to study her face, and to contemplate what's going on behind that furrowed newborn brow.

New babies have a wise look. Maybe it's because they really do know a lot. Don't let anyone tell you differently. Friends, relatives, and caregivers will say things like "Oh, she's only a newborn, she can't do anything yet," "They don't really see anything at this age, do they?", "That's not a smile, that's just gas," "Sleep and eat, that's all they do." But they're wrong.

Your newborn is a fascinating person, and not just to her proud, star-struck, ecstatic parents. Studies have shown that newborns really can see, hear, taste, smell, feel, and think. Many of your newborn's amazing abilities help her to get attached to her mother—to you. Getting attached means not only getting to know and trust you, but also drawing you hopelessly into her power. Newborns come equipped to make their parents fall in love with them.

Newborn babies' favorite thing to look at is a human face. They see most clearly at a distance of eight to twelve inches, the space between an infant's face and her mother's during

Even if you find baby talk embarrassing, you may soon find yourself chattering away in singsong Motherese. As you do, your baby is learning another way to connect with you.

breastfeeding. Within a few weeks your baby will have enough control over her eyes to gaze steadily into your eyes, and she'll prefer your face to that of a stranger.

Tiny babies can hear as well as or better than adults. But they are more sensitive to sound, and when awake they often startle at loud noises. They find high-pitched, feminine voices to be the most soothing; by the time a baby is twenty to thirty days old she can tell her mother's voice from that of a stranger. They also have an amazing capacity to block out sounds from their environment; they can fall asleep to the sound of the vacuum cleaner or loud music on the stereo. In fact, if the noise around a newborn is too much for her senses, sleep is her way of escape.

Newborns even respond to the changing rhythms and sounds of language. In face-to-face "conversation," they move in synchrony with their mothers' speech. This "dance" is very subtle; researchers discovered it by analyzing video tapes frame by frame. Even if you find baby talk embarrassing, you may soon find yourself chattering away in singsong Motherese. As you do, your baby is learning another way to connect with you. She watches your lips and your eyes move, and she is fascinated. Your baby is already learning about talking, and she's only a few days old.

As for taste and smell, babies come into this world prepared to like their mother's sweet milk. Their sense of smell guides them right to it. When babies only a few days old were each presented with two breast pads, one from the baby's own mother and one from another nursing mother, each turned her head toward the scent of her personal food source. If you hold your tiny newborn in your arms when she's hungry, she'll turn and squirm and try to move herself right to where the milk is (though she'll be confused about where to aim her mouth if you touch her cheek or even the back of her head).

Do tiny babies feel things? They know when they feel hungry, and they know what to do about it. Their mouths open, their heads turn from side to side, searching for a nipple. Maybe they find their fists instead, but chewing on a fist won't do for long. These early hunger signals from your baby will quickly escalate to a cry, until you pick your baby up and feed her. Heed the early hunger signals, and your baby won't have to cry. She'll stay calmer and will be easier to feed, and you'll have taught her that she doesn't have to get herself all frazzled just to have her needs met.

The best time to study your baby is when she is in the state of "quiet-alert." She's awake, her eyes are open, and she's relatively still. This is when a newborn is at her most magical. Most newborns spend the first hour or so after birth in the quiet-alert state, which is why they should be with their parents during this time—not in bassinets by themselves. Periods of quiet-alert won't last as long in the days to come, though they will gradually lengthen as your baby learns from you how to keep herself under control. When you see your baby wide-eyed and quietly looking around, take the time to enjoy her. Later you can talk to visitors or finish your lunch.

Follow your heart as you get to know your new child. Because you care about your baby more than anyone, it is you who will do the best job of figuring out what she's doing and feeling and what she needs. "Experts" such as nursery nurses and grandmas may swoop down upon you and try to tell you what to do. Some of their advice may be valuable, but you are the expert on your own baby. The bond between the two of you has been growing for many months already.

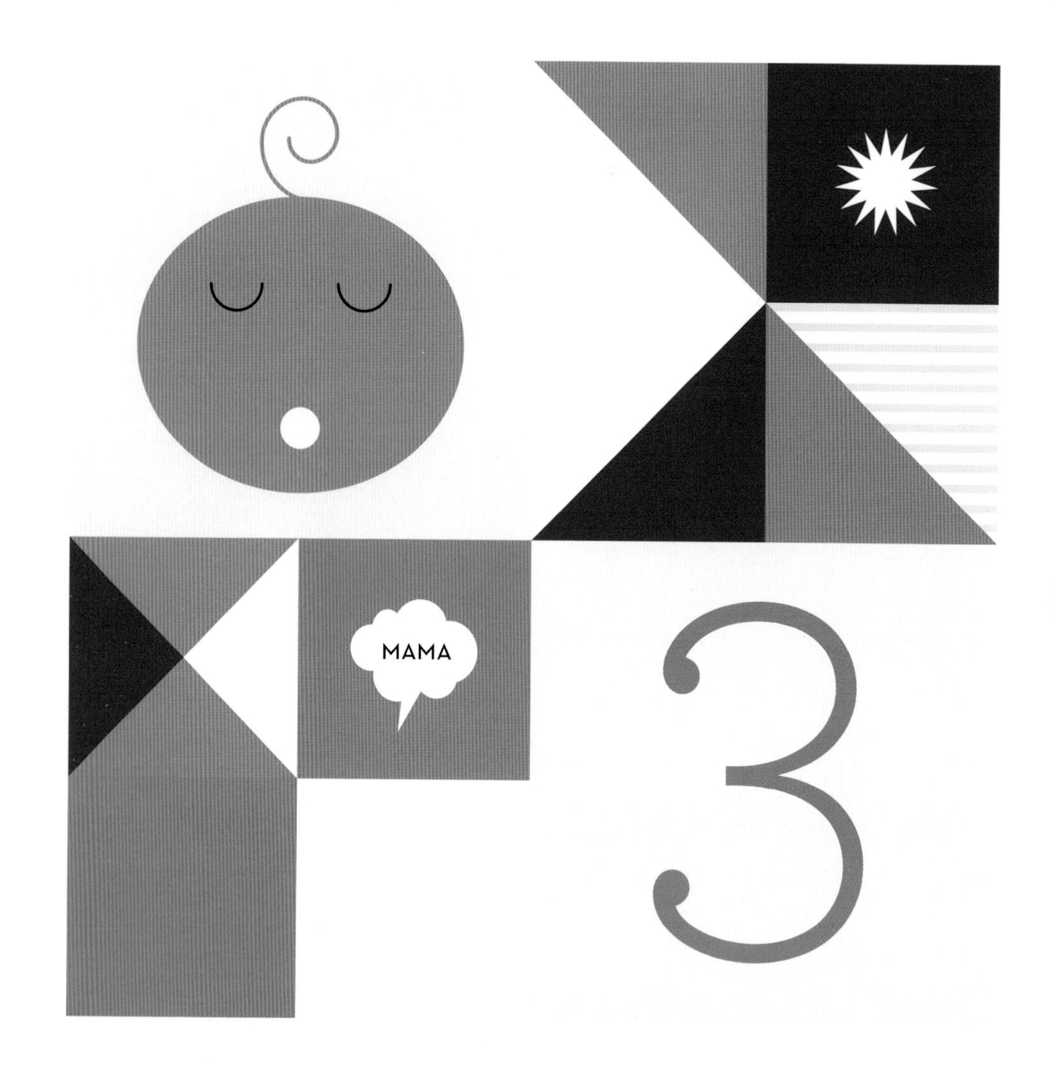
MAMA
3

You and Your Baby Need to Stay Together

Imagine that you're a baby in the womb, soon to be born. What's your world like? There's not much to see—maybe some dim light filters through if Mom is standing in bright sunlight without too much clothing on. There's more to hear—muffled voices from the outside, some of them familiar, some good music if you're lucky, the occasional loud noise that makes you jump, and the steady background sounds of the placenta swishing blood back and forth, and of Mom's body, her heartbeat, her breathing, maybe some rumblings from her tummy.

But what do you feel? Always warm, held and caressed by the firm muscles of Mom's uterus. You are lulled into sleep by the motions of your mother's body, surrounded by the soft touch of the amniotic fluid you float in, relatively weightless. You don't know what it is to be hungry or thirsty, since you are fed at a constant rate through the umbilical cord and can take a drink from that constant supply of lovely fluid.

Now imagine that you've just been born. You get a crash course in breathing, and then suddenly there are things to see. But everything is so painfully bright that you quickly learn to keep your eyes shut till someone turns down the lights. Noises are louder, especially the newest sound of all—your own crying, which is pretty darn scary. Your arms and legs move freely in the open air, and that's scary, too. You're happier if someone holds onto them for you so you can stop being startled into crying harder. There's more going on in your world than you've ever had to cope with before. In small doses it's fascinating, but mostly it's frightening because it's all so new and so very different.

Where do you want to be? You can't go back into Mom's womb. What's the next best thing? This plastic box you're in now, with the hard, flat mattress that doesn't move? At least the blanket is warm, but it feels rough on your tender skin. There is

These first special days of your baby's life are a time not to be missed—there's too much to learn and savor!

a lot of arm and leg room, certainly, but that's hardly what you need—you're used to being curled up inside Mom's uterus. How about that nurse over there? She's coming to pick you up. Feels okay—but that voice is not one you recognize. She's looking at the clock. Uh-oh, time for her to go home. You long for a secure place to stay and someone you can count on.

How about Mom? She kept you safe when you were inside her. Can she help you out now? She can hold you close and help you control those limbs that seem to have a life of their own. Her skin next to yours feels soooo soft and warm. You can suck at her breasts, and that's what really calms you down after that wild and scary entrance you just made. Her movements feel awfully familiar—you feel soothed by the way her chest moves in and out rhythmically, and when she moves her whole body you understand it all from the outside now. If she holds you just so, so your ear is against her chest, you hear something that you can really grab on to—that heartbeat rhythm you know so well. Now you can open your eyes a little longer because Mom got somebody to dim those glaring lights, and you get the reward of a lifetime—two beautiful eyes meeting yours. You get lost in those round dark pools of love light. You decide this new place is a definite improvement over that plastic box. Eventually you discover that familiar swaying movement when she carries you around or rocks in the rocking chair. The motion lulls you right to sleep. It's a lot like being back in the womb again, maybe even better. This could be just what you need to help you get your life together as a newly born person. . . .

Babies belong with their mothers. This simple truth seems obvious to me, as it may to you, too. Certainly it's clear that new babies are most comfortable when they are held a lot, rather than left to lie somewhere on their own. If they are put down they need their mothers to respond to them quickly, before they're crying so hard that even getting what they need won't calm them down. They need to be fed often—every two to three hours—and they sometimes like a little snack in between, which

How a mother and baby get started with each other makes a difference.

When a mother brings her newborn in for a two-week checkup, I can often tell whether or not she roomed-in with her baby. Rooming-in mothers exude more confidence, less worry. They seem to be more in sync with their babies, better able to read and respond to their baby's cues. Not only does their milk appear sooner, but rooming-in mothers experience fewer breastfeeding problems. It's important for the newborn to know right away to whom he belongs, and for the new mother not to leave the hospital a stranger to her baby.

—Bill

is easy since the breasts are so handy. They need to be close to that familiar heartbeat. They need someone to understand how very frightening it is to feel hunger, to experience stillness, and to be left alone—to understand how new and different all this is. They need to be held until they fall sound asleep, and many people, including me, believe they need to sleep next to their mothers.

What may not be so obvious is how much mothers need to be with their babies. You have a lot to teach your baby, and also a lot to learn from him. Mastering these lessons in your first few weeks together will make the months to come much easier for both of you. Right from the start, you can help your baby feel that the world is a pretty nice place to be, and that he can trust you to keep it that way. If you're right there to soothe him when he fusses, he won't get much practice at full-blown howling, and he'll be easier to live with because he knows that help is only a whimper away. You'll teach him to be happy, and he'll teach you how to feel needed.

Breastfeeding will go more smoothly if you have unlimited opportunities to practice in the first days after birth. At first, your baby gets a nice, soft nipple on which to perfect his sucking skills, along with a lot of colostrum to protect him from illness. When your actual milk is ready and plentiful, he'll be an eager expert, capable of getting much of that milk out, so you'll have fewer problems with engorgement.

Ask for 24-hour rooming-in while you're in the hospital. Don't worry that this will be too much of a strain on you; the reverse could actually be true. Most mothers rest better knowing their babies are close by and content. Your baby will have a head start on getting tuned in to your sleeping and waking cycles if he's away from the 24-hour bright lights and bustle of the hospital nursery. You yourself may actually get better care from the nursing staff if you room in; if you're taking care of the baby, the nurses have no one to fuss over but you. Even if you've had a cesarean, you should still be able to keep your baby with you. Dad, Grandma, or (occasionally) a nurse can give you a hand when you need it. It's best to plan for someone to stay with you full time.

These first special days of your baby's life are a time not to be missed—there's too much to learn and savor! Keep your baby with you as much as possible while you're in the hospital. You'll go home with a happy baby, and you'll already feel confident as a mother.

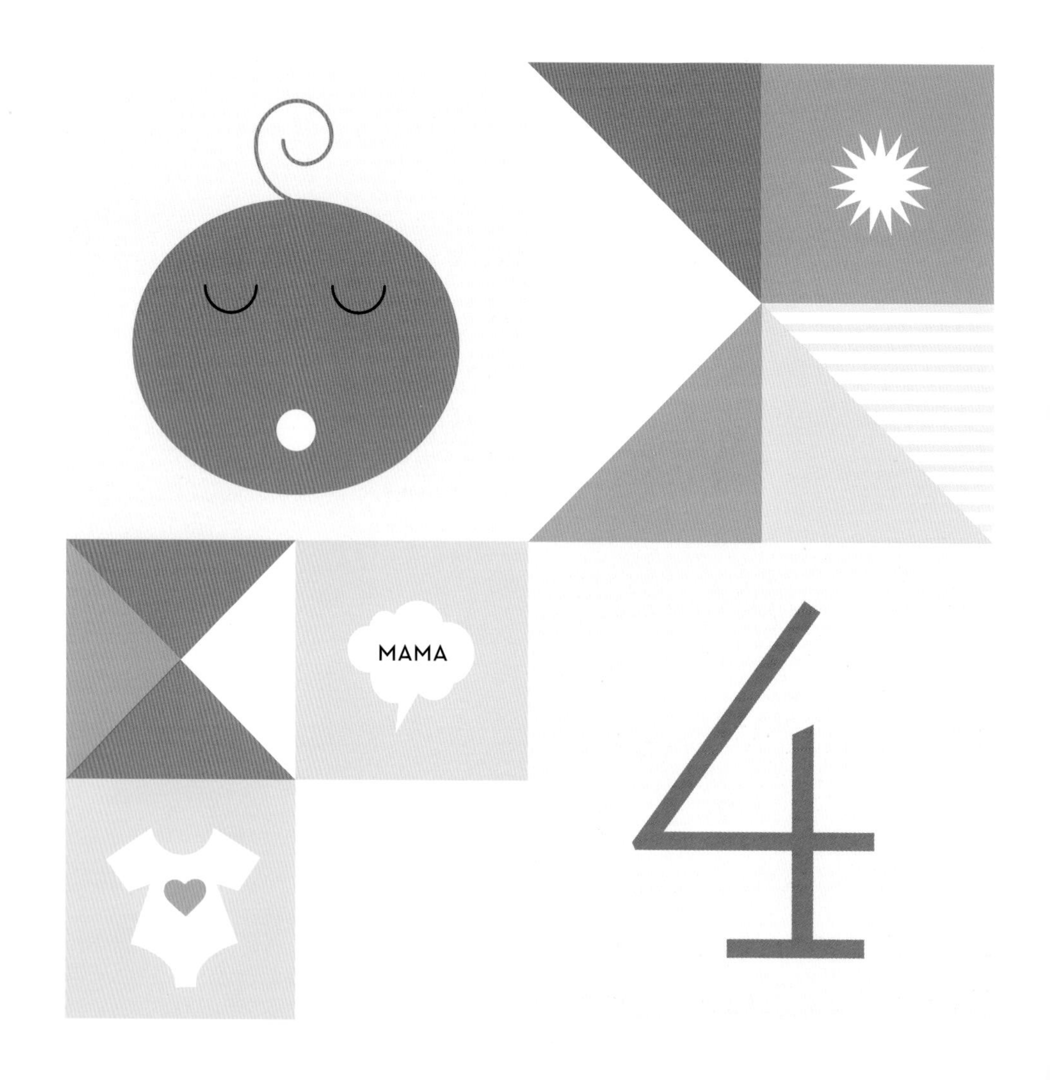
MAMA
4

Breastfeeding Really Is Better Than Bottle-Feeding

I could make a very long list of good reasons for breastfeeding your baby. It would include headings like "perfect nutrition," "protection from illness," "brain growth," "long-term health benefits," and "psychological advantages." You'd find items such as "less risk of Sudden Infant Death Syndrome" and "fewer ear infections."

But how does this translate into *your* life with your baby? Will you really see a difference if you breastfeed?

The answer is "Absolutely." And the advantages will be apparent in a lot of ways.

Let's start with a matter that is very close to home—how your baby smells. Breastfed babies, even ones with a tendency to spit up, smell better than their formula-fed counterparts. If the baby spits up on your shoulder, your shirt may smell a little sour after an hour or two, but spit-up breast milk doesn't smell nearly as bad as spit-up formula, and spit-up milk washes out easily without leaving stains as formula does. And because breast milk is easier to digest than formula, breastfed babies' stools have only a "cheesy" sort of smell that is not offensive. This makes diaper changing more appealing to Dad as well as Mom.

Here's another advantage that goes beyond the scientific. When you breastfeed, you always have a close-at-hand method available for comforting and quieting your baby, a maternal secret weapon that comes in handy when you're around people who have a low tolerance for infant crying (and that includes just about everybody). Sucking soothes infants, even when they're not hungry. The rhythm of the suck, the closeness to Mom, the trickle of milk all help to restore the baby's feeling of rightness. When you're breastfeeding, you don't have to go hunting for the pacifier when your baby is fussy. (If your baby doesn't want to suck she'll let you know—sometimes babies just want to be held while they have a good cry.)

You also don't have to worry about overfeeding a breastfed baby. Studies show that babies have a remarkable ability to fine-tune their intake of breast milk, all on their own. The infant's way of sucking regulates how much milk she gets, and if she is only sucking for comfort she won't get a full meal. All you have to do is offer your breast, and then put your feet up and relax. Breastfeeding is the original convenience food.

Some babies do take more milk than they need. But if your baby is eating too much, she'll spit up milk and you'll know to try other ways of comforting. If she still insists on sucking, give her just one breast at a feeding, and wait three hours before beginning to use the other breast. Use the "empty" breast for between-feed snacks.

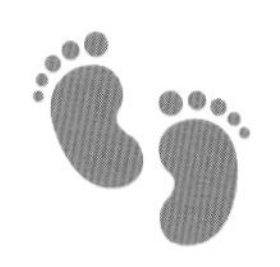

No new mother likes to think about her perfect little one coming down with a cold or flu, but that miserable first cold or tummy ache is inevitable. Breastfeeding will make it easier. First of all, breastfed babies really do get sick less. You may wait a lot longer for that first sniffle, and your baby is far less likely to become really sick. Stomach flu may be mowing down

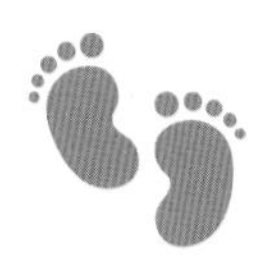

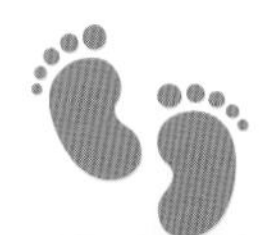

family members one by one, but the breastfed baby might well escape the family bug. Second, if your baby is feeling a little under the weather, her more frequent demands to feed ensure that she gets the fluids she needs and help her stay comfortable, and maybe even a little more cheerful. Having a healthier baby really enhances your mothering. It's so much easier to be a happy mother to someone who is behaving pleasantly, and having a way to make an unhappy baby feel better makes you feel more competent and confident.

My list of reasons for breastfeeding would also include a heading about breastfeeding being better for mothers. Breastfeeding will help you lose the weight you gained in pregnancy, and you won't have to go on a restricted diet to do so. Nursing lowers your chances of getting breast cancer. For the first six months, provided your baby is exclusively breastfed (using no pacifiers, bottles, or solids) and you haven't menstruated, your risk of getting pregnant again is less than 2 percent—comparable to rates cited for various methods of artificial birth control.

Then there's the matter of what breastfeeding can do for your mothering. La Leche League, the breastfeeding support organization, used to have a slogan on its stationery proclaiming "Good mothering through breastfeeding." Some people felt

Studies show that babies have a remarkable ability to fine-tune their intake of breast milk, all on their own. All you have to do is offer your breast, and then put your feet up and relax.

that these words implied that women who bottle-feed must be bad mothers, but this isn't how the slogan was in-tended to be understood. What it meant is that breastfeeding leads to good mothering—it's a way of becoming a good mother to your baby.

Biology is closely linked to behavior when you breastfeed. In order for your body to produce the amount of milk your baby needs to thrive, you must recognize and respond to her hunger cues. So breastfeeding forces you to really get to know your baby. Breastfed newborns need to feed often—eight, ten, even twelve times a day. Each feeding time is an opportunity for interaction, for touching, and for enjoying each other, things that build the bond between you and your baby. Yes, of course, bottle-feeding mothers can do these things during feedings, too, but they happen automatically during breastfeeding. This is one of the ways our biology helps ensure that each baby has someone who really cares about what happens to her.

Breastfeeding affects biology in ways beyond your milk supply. The skin-to-skin contact probably helps to reduce stress reactions in mother and baby alike. More impressively, the two hormones that are associated with milk production and the re-lease of the milk (prolactin and oxytocin, respectively) help you to have good feelings about your baby. Prolactin is associated with feelings of calm, and in some animals it regulates mothering behavior. Oxytocin, too, produces pleasant emotions and contributes to the formation of bonds between human beings. It is released during sexual intercourse and in labor, as well as during breastfeeding sessions. After noting oxytocin's role in these three intense interpersonal acts, one wise researcher dubbed oxytocin "the hormone of love."

You will notice a feeling of relaxation coming over you as you feed your baby—perhaps not in the first few days when both of you are learning what to do, but soon. Sitting down to relax and breastfeed your baby can release tension and even lull you into one of those naps that new mothers need but may be reluctant to take.

Breastfeeding is a joy, an experience not to be missed. It may not fill you with profound wisdom. You may not have brilliant insight about the meaning of life while you're nursing (though you may find yourself thinking about it). But nursing will help you fall in love with your baby and feel proud of yourself as well.

MAMA
5

You Can Solve Breastfeeding Problems

So you've heard that breastfeeding is not so simple? That some mothers just don't have enough milk (see Chapter 21, page 165, on that subject)? That sore nipples are not just sore, they're excruciating? That your breasts will leak, you will smell like a dairy, and you will feel like a cow? That some babies are barracudas—ouch!—and others just don't take to it? You've heard that there's a down side to breastfeeding?

Perhaps there is, for some women, but these problems can almost always be prevented or solved. For example, you don't have to put up with sore nipples. They're not inevitable. Nipples get sore when babies aren't latching on properly. During breastfeeding, your nipple is supposed to be far back in the baby's mouth, where it can't get hurt. If the baby doesn't get enough breast tissue in his mouth, the nipple ends up in the front of the mouth, where the motion of the jaws and the tongue can damage the nipple's tender skin. Some babies latch on like experts from the first suck, but most need some guidance so they'll get it right. One of your first jobs as a mother is to teach your baby the right way to latch on and suck, so that your nipples won't get sore. If you're reading this too late to avoid sore nipples, then you'll know what to do to get them to heal quickly.

Breastfeeding is not terribly difficult, but it doesn't come entirely naturally, either. These early days are a learning period for you and your baby. Eventually your baby will be able to latch on to the breast without either of you giving it a thought, but in these first feeding sessions you need to pay attention to what he is doing. You should not let him latch on and suck however he happens to, not if this is causing you pain. Breastfeeding shouldn't hurt.

Breastfeeding shouldn't hurt.

Here's a brief lesson in proper positioning. First, get comfortable yourself. Sitting up in a chair with arms is usually easiest. Put a pillow under your elbow on the side that will be holding the baby, and another on your lap to bring the baby up level with your nipple. The pillows support you, so that you can relax and not strain your muscles as you hold your baby. Use a footstool (or a stack of books) under your feet to raise your lap.

Hold your baby in the cradle of your arm, his neck by the end of your elbow, your hand grasping his bottom. This is called the cradle hold. The baby should be turned on his side, facing you, tummy to tummy. His head and neck should be straight, not turned sideways and not arched back. The pillow supports your arm as you cradle the baby up close to your chest. Don't leave this job to your muscles; if you do, they will get tired. As the baby slips down, your nipple will be stretched and pulled to the front of the baby's mouth, where it can get hurt.

If you're having problems getting at your baby's mouth because his arms are flailing around his face, tuck the bottom arm between his body and your squishy stomach (see, it's good for something!). Try to hold his upper arm down with the thumb of your hand that holds the baby's bottom. The hand that isn't holding the baby supports your breast—fingers underneath, thumb on top (well behind the areola, the darker area around the nipple).

Now comes the most important part: getting the baby onto the breast correctly. Express a little colostrum or milk onto the nipple just to get the baby interested. Tickle his lips gently with the nipple to encourage him to open his mouth wide, as in a yawn. When you see his mouth open very wide, direct your nipple into the center of it, and, with your arm, quickly pull him in close to you so that he gets a large mouthful of breast, including at least an inch of the areola. This is important, because the sinuses where the milk is stored are under the areola; the baby's gums must compress these sinuses to get milk out. If he sucks only on the nipple, he will not get much milk, and you will get very sore.

The baby's lips should be flanged outward during feedings (have a nurse show you the "fish lips" look by pulling down on the lower lip and flipping up the upper lip); and the tip of his nose should touch the breast. He can still breathe this way, from the sides of his nostrils, but if his nose seems to be blocked, you can change his position slightly by pulling his bottom in closer to you. As he starts to suck, you should see movement all the way back to his ears, as his jaws work to get milk from the breast. You should also hear swallowing.

Does all this sound terribly complicated? Are you wondering where you'll get a third hand to hold these instructions while you are working with your baby? Relax—breastfeeding is simpler than it sounds. And if you don't get it right the first time (you'll know because it will hurt), just try again. Take the baby off the breast—break the suction first, by wedging a finger into his mouth between his gums—and once again tickle his lips with the nipple. Getting it right may take several tries, and that's okay. Consider this to be a good practice and an investment in a happy breastfeeding relationship in the days to come. Do your best to stay calm and relaxed yourself—put on some

Perhaps the reason some women choose not to breastfeed or do not persevere in overcoming a rough start is that they are not fully convinced breastfeeding makes a difference.

After decades of experience as a parent and babywatcher, I can truly say breastfeeding matters. You can look at every system in the baby's body and see the benefits of human milk for human babies: Breast milk is better for vision and oral development; breastfed babies have fewer ear infections; breast milk is more physiologic for the cardiovascular system and kidneys; intestinal immunity is enhanced by human milk; breast milk is ideal for cholesterol metabolism; and, last but not least, breast milk enhances intelligence. My wish as a pediatrician is that mothers value breastfeeding for all it is worth and do not just consider it an optional way of feeding their babies.

—Bill

soft music and don't feel you have to rush. If the baby gets upset during feeding sessions, pause for a while and calm him down before returning to the lesson. If you start to get frustrated, take a few deep breaths and remember that you're the mother here. It's your job even now to guide your child in the way he should go. Learning to breastfeed correctly is his first experience with your loving, disciplinary guidance.

I've included this information about latching on because it is important to be able to get breastfeeding off to a good start. Your careful attention now to positioning and latch-on technique will prevent problems in the days to come, problems that would make it less enjoyable for you to nurse your baby. If things are not going well, consult a lactation specialist in the first few days of breastfeeding. Your baby should be seen by a health-care provider *in person* four or five days after leaving the hospital to be sure breastfeeding is going well, even if you are not worried, and even if the baby has had a complete medical exam two to three days after birth.

You'll get a lot of advice as a breastfeeding mother. Some of it will be useful, and some of it may send you down the path toward early weaning before you know this is happening. So that you can tell the difference between the good and bad, learn all you can about breastfeeding ahead of time. Attend at least one La Leche League meeting. Read *The Breastfeeding Book* (see Resources, page 204). If you have a problem, seek help from a League leader (to find a good one, call 877-452-5324 or visit their Web site at www.lalecheleague.org) or a lactation consultant. Most breastfeeding problems *can* be solved.

MAMA
6

New Mothers Need Special Care

Societies all around the world have ways of taking care of new mothers. There may be a special place for them to stay, certain foods they are to eat or avoid, rules about when they can leave their beds, go outside, or return to their usual work. Not all of these customs make a lot of sense outside of the cultures in which they originate, but all of these societies agree on one thing—new mothers need to be cared for.

This is very wise, and we sophisticated, capable, 21st-century liberated women should take note. We like to think that we, like our hearty peasant ancestors, should be able to come in from the field just long enough to have our babies and then get back out there and finish hoeing the row we were working on before the labor pains overwhelmed us. This is really wrongheaded. The truth is, our peasant ancestors didn't do it this way—and neither should we. We owe ourselves and our babies a better start than this in our new life together.

One of the best things you can do for your new baby is to take care of your baby's mother. Don't take this responsibility lightly. This is a stressful time for you, and being well rested, well fed, and unharried will help you cope with the changes and demands of your new life.

Getting enough rest may be the biggest challenge new mothers face. Newborns know nothing about adult sleep needs. They stay up until midnight. They wake up twice in the night to be fed. Then they sleep the whole next day, it seems. Tomorrow's pattern may be completely different from yesterday's. This all adds up to quite a change from the bed-at-eleven, rise-at-seven routine that adults are accustomed to follow.

The birth itself may leave you feeling sleep-deprived, especially if you labored all night or went into labor after only a few hours of sleep. Immediately after your baby is born, you may experience a "high" that keeps you awake, but this feeling will end with a yawn and a crash. Unfortunately, hospital routines may keep you from getting the rest you need, so that you go home feeling tired.

A wise mother soon learns to nap whenever she can. Newborns often fall into a deep sleep an hour or two after birth, and this should be your first cue to get some rest yourself. Once you get home from the hospital, try to sleep when the baby sleeps during the day. Relax on your bed with your little one cuddled up next to you or even lying on your chest. It's a wonderful feeling to share such peace with this little person who so recently was inside you, kicking and keeping you awake at bedtime. (See Chapter 10 to learn more about safety precautions for sharing sleep with your baby.) That extra hour or two of sleep during the day will make it much easier for you to be patient when your baby awakens in the middle of the night. Even a 20-minute catnap can perk you up when you're still tired from the night before. Napping is one of the hidden joys of motherhood; you'll find yourself longing for naps long after your children have stopped taking them.

Try to take it easy during your first weeks of motherhood. Don't get dressed; take a shower and put on a fresh nursing gown or something to lounge in. Put on street clothes only for taking walks. This reminds you and everyone else that you're off duty except for baby care. Put your feet up. Read a good book. Limit visitors, both the number and the length of time they stay.

There is one kind of visitor that you and your family need in the days after birth, and that is the kind that does housework. If you can afford to hire help, pay someone (or several helpers) to clean, cook, run errands, and entertain the baby's older siblings. This is a much smarter investment than hiring a baby nurse. You should be the one caring for your baby, not some stiff-uniformed expert who isn't even related to her.

Friends, Grandmas, and other family members can all help out with these tasks, freeing you to concentrate on your baby. You have to let these helpers know what your needs are and that their role is to take care of Mom. They can bring meals, clean up, shop for groceries, do the laundry. Never turn down even a casual offer of help. Practice saying, "Could you bring dinner?" or "Would you mind folding and putting away a load of laundry?" so that the words come easily to mind when someone asks, "Is there anything I can do?" It's your right as a new mother to sit still and hold your baby, while everyone else fusses over you and your household. Don't forget that new fathers

Limit visitors, both the number and the length of time they stay.

need special care and rest, too; encourage your husband to take as much time off work as possible, and get friends to help, if you can, so that Dad doesn't have to do all the housework.

Another type of helper you might consider hiring is a postpartum doula. *Doula* is a Greek word that means "woman's servant." Doulas are trained to provide support for women and their families during labor and the postpartum period. A postpartum doula can assist you with breastfeeding and learning to care for your baby. She will provide support and companionship in a manner that boosts your mothering confidence. She can also help your spouse and other family members figure out how they can best help you. (See Resources, page 202, for contact information for Doulas of North America [DONA]. This organization can help you find a doula in your area.)

Do take some time for yourself every day. Soak in the tub or take a long shower. Fix your hair. Find something comfortable to wear that looks nice (easier said than done in the first weeks postpartum—how about sweats in a pretty color or leggings and a big print top?). Rent a favorite video to watch while the baby nurses. Indulge in your favorite carry-out food.

Relax, enjoy, and don't feel guilty about being pampered. You're doing all these things for your baby's mother, which means that you're also doing them for your baby.

MAMA
7

All Your Energy Goes to the Baby

In the days before you had a baby, did you ever spend time with friends who had just become parents? Do you remember noticing that they could talk of nothing else but their baby? Were you puzzled at how one tiny creature, who did little besides sleep, eat, and cry or fuss, could take over adult lives so completely?

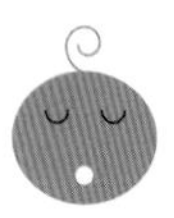

Parenting a new baby is an intense experience. It's joyful, it's scary, it's time-consuming.

Now you know.

Parenting a new baby is an intense experience. It's joyful, it's scary, it's time-consuming. For a while, at least, all your energy must go toward the baby. You learn on the job, and you're on the job all the time. You want to do everything you're supposed to, everything you can to help your baby be healthy and happy. This is no small task to set for yourself, and, as with any big goal or dream, reaching it takes commitment.

Emotional adjustments are an intense part of new parenthood. You feel a fierce attachment to your baby, but it may not be quite what you expected mother-love to be. Your self-image is altered by motherhood, and the changes you are going through may threaten at times to overwhelm everything you thought you knew about yourself.

Why do you have these intense feelings about the baby and motherhood? First of all, this baby was recently residing in your body. Because of this, you may feel a oneness with your baby, as if the two of you are actually one person. If the baby is upset, therefore, you feel the same way, not just in sympathy or frustration, but because you and the baby still share emotions. If the baby tenses his muscles, you will tighten yours, too. If the baby is having trouble with breastfeeding or has some kind of medical problem, you take it personally—something that's wrong with your baby is also wrong with you. Your baby experiences this oneness even more intensely. It will be many months before the baby knows that he is a human being separate from you, with his own individual vantage point on life.

Your relationship with your baby and your adjustment to motherhood also depend on how you yourself were mothered. Feelings of fear, frustration, and abandonment left over from when you were an infant can intensify your empathy with your baby and make it harder for you to hang on to your sense of grown-up identity, the part of you that says you are now the responsible mother and no longer the infant.

It helps to know to what degree your needs as a baby were met. If you were not responded to quickly as a young baby and were left alone a lot to cry—and when your mother did respond it was in a distant, detached, or inconsistent way—you will have more intense feelings when your baby needs you. This intensity can cause you to either shut down your intuition and fail to respond quickly and warmly or to respond almost desperately to protect your baby from feeling so fearful and abandoned. If you recognize this in yourself you may find that as you mother your baby in a responsive way you are also mothering that frightened baby inside you. This insight can help you develop a perspective on the intense emotions you experience, such as deep guilt when you can't seem to comfort your baby or extreme frustration or anger when your own needs have to be put aside.

Other stresses in your life can take your energy away from the baby. These might include problems in your marriage, criticism from your mother or mother-in-law, financial or career pressures, a move, or major remodeling. Any of these things can disturb your mental peace and affect your maternal emotions. If for some reason you are not feeling good about yourself, it will be hard for you to feel good about your baby. For a while, at least, you need to minimize the demands and worries that divert energy away from your baby.

Even everyday problems may be too distracting at this time. This is why women who have just had babies need to be cared for. With all your energy going to building your relationship with the baby and learning your new role as a mother, you may have no energy left over to worry about dust on the living room furniture or about what Aunt Matilda thinks of your mothering.

Whether a hired helper, a family member, a friend, or your husband, someone should have the job of caring for you so that you can care for your baby. Be clear about this with your helpers. If the baby's grandmother has come to visit, be sure she knows ahead of time that her main job is to take care of the household while your job is to take care of the baby. I hear stories of how visitors come for two weeks and expect to be waited on, while also criticizing how things are done. Taking care of you also means running interference with people who cause tension, a job that caring husbands are especially well suited for.

Your newborn infant has an intense need for you right now. You are the comforting one and the connecting one. You have the familiar voice, the smell, the rhythm, the milk—all the

In their zeal to meet their babies' needs, many new mothers often neglect their own needs.

Even Martha, an experienced mother of eight, is guilty of this overgiving. In fact, it is the most committed mothers who are prone to burnout, since you first have to be "on fire" in order to burn out. As a caring mate and father, I have learned to intervene when Martha says, "The baby needs me so much, I don't even have time to take a shower." I gently respond, "Martha, what our baby needs is a rested and happy mother." One of the most important gifts you can give your baby is to mirror a happy face. If you are tired, stressed, and not meeting your own needs, you will not mirror happiness to your baby, and the whole family loses. I have had to remind Martha to take care of herself so that she could take better care of our babies.

—Bill

things he needs to feel secure. No one else, not even the baby's father, can fill your shoes. The extent of your responsibility may seem staggering at first. Even when you're sleeping you are listening for your infant. When you're awake he is in your arms, and much of that time he is feeding. Has anything in your life prepared you for being on call 24 hours of every day? Even a challenging, high-paying job can't equip you for the awesome load of having somebody be so totally dependent upon you.

At times you will feel that you need a break from your baby, just to catch your breath and regain your balance. I'm all in favor of time-outs for new mothers, opportunities to take a short walk or a bath while someone else holds the baby, but these breaks should be short ones, just long enough to refresh and collect yourself. Most of the time in the first months postpartum you should keep your baby close to you, because he himself is the best cure for your doubts and uncertainties as a mother. Every time you feed, comfort, hold, or nap with your baby you are improving your mothering skills and strengthening your bond. You are learning to interpret your baby's cues, and you are also getting positive reinforcement from your baby's soft skin, his skill at the breast, his contentment while he sleeps.

Taking charge of your baby will help you understand where you leave off and he begins. You don't want to lose your empathy for your baby, but you do want to become the one your baby trusts to make hunger go away, the one whose loving arms tenderly support a body that is still unsure of where it is in space. As you become more practiced at reading your baby's cues and helping him regulate his behavior, you will feel less frantic when he fusses. Knowing that you can usually make the crying end will lessen your own feelings of helplessness.

Putting all this energy into your baby in his first weeks of life will teach him to trust you, and you will discover that you can trust yourself as a mother. The months ahead will be much easier because you have dealt with this intense time of change directly, getting to know your baby and yourself as his mother, rather than letting other people take charge and much less important matters distract you. Doing this hard work in the beginning will save you from having much harder work to do as your child grows up.

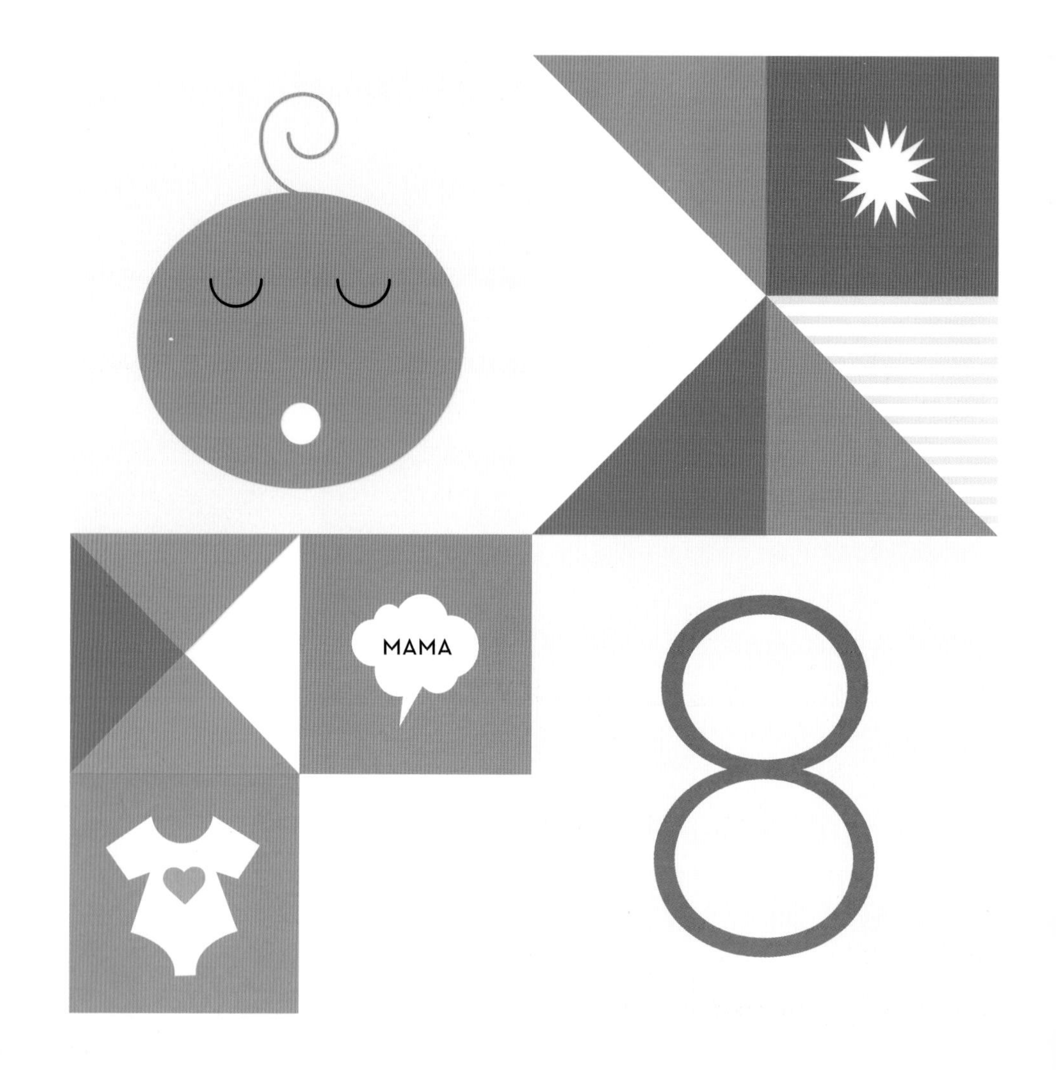
MAMA
8

Your Baby Needs Your Help When She Cries

Cries are a baby's language. They are her most direct, most urgent way of communicating with you. If she called out, "Mama, come help me," wouldn't you rush to her side? Crying calls for the same kind of response, and while you can't make her stop crying, you can help her to calm down and pull herself back together.

If you're like most mothers, you really can't stand to hear your baby cry. This is the way it's supposed to be. A baby's cry has that compelling, gotta-do-something-about-it quality to ensure that the baby gets taken care of, preferably right away. Often, just picking her up, walking with her, talking or humming, and rubbing her back will quiet her quickly. Offering the breast works also. Many mothers intuitively know that holding and nursing keeps a baby content, so they just do that and avoid a lot of crying (see Chapter 9, page 77).

Even though a crying baby needs her mother's comfort, it's important to remember that you are not the reason your baby cries, nor do you have to stop the cries. Babies cry because of their own inner needs and their individual temperaments. Some cry more and harder than others even when they are being held (though being held more may reduce the crying). They do this not because their parents are less capable, but because the babies have come wired that way. Remembering this can help you stay calm when your baby is very fussy. It's not your fault that your baby is crying, but it is your job to help and support her until she feels better.

You may also need to do some research on the cause of the crying if holding and nursing are not working. First, of course, you should have the baby checked by a doctor. This may not help, though; as we have discussed in *The Baby Book* (see

Resources, page 204), many doctors fail to recognize certain physical problems as possible causes of a baby's crying. One of these causes is gastroesophageal reflux; another is the breastfeeding mother's diet. My sixth baby, at two weeks, began crying inconsolably in my arms. He refused my breast and was obviously in pain. I had been counseling other mothers to eliminate dairy products from their diets for this same behavior, and now it was my turn to "go off dairy." Because he was so gassy and in such intense pain, I went one step further. I went on what's known as the Caveman Diet (see Resources, page 206) and the crying stopped within two days.

Responding to your baby's cries is one of the most important things you do in the early months. When you pay attention to her cries, you are teaching your baby things that are very important for her healthy development. When you respond to your baby's cries, she learns that she can make things happen. She is an important person, someone whose complaints matter. She learns that the world of her family is a loving place, where there are people who help her feel good. As you help her calm down, she discovers that distress is followed by comfort. All of these lessons decrease her inner anxiety, and she gets in the habit of feeling peaceful most of the time.

If you respond promptly to your baby's cries in the early days, within a month or two she will most likely be crying a lot

If you respond to the early fussing noises, you can usually get the baby back into a peaceful mood fairly easily.

less. This is a big advantage for you; it's much easier to mother a happy baby. Quick responses to your baby's cries also prevent here from getting into a real frenzy of crying, the kind that is hard to get her out of. If you respond to the early fussing noises, you can usually get the baby back into a peaceful mood fairly easily. If you wait until the fussing escalates into full-blown howling, you'll have to spend a lot more time calming the baby. She'll be angry and trembling and may continue to sob for a long time. All that needless hard crying will also leave you feeling tense and shaken, even guilty—it's hard not to when those little eyes look at you so helplessly. Whatever time you may have gained for yourself by not responding to the early noises is lost in the time it takes to get everyone feeling content again.

The baby who receives an early response to her cries learns that all she has to do is fuss a little and someone comes to help her. Does this mean she's spoiled? Not at all. It means that she is learning to use subtle cues to get her needs met. Pretty soon, her mother will know her so well that she may not even have to fuss. For example, Mom knows that Baby likes to be picked up right when she awakens, so Mom goes to her as soon as she hears waking sounds on the intercom. Baby comes to trust that Mom will be there at the end of a nap, so Baby doesn't waste energy becoming frightened. Both Mom and Baby feel good about understanding each other so well.

Waiting to pick up a crying baby teaches different lessons. First, she learns that nobody listens to her unless she cries hard. So when she needs her mother's presence she doesn't waste much time on subtle openings. She just lets loose. If time after time nobody comes to help her, she may eventually learn not to cry; the reason she stops signaling her parents is because she has given up. She knows it won't do any good. This does not leave her feeling right inside, and it teaches her not to trust her parents. Her mother might congratulate herself on how content her baby is to play alone, but she and the baby feel more like neighbors or acquaintances, not like family members who care about what is going on inside each other.

When your baby is new, don't bother debating with yourself about how soon to pick her up when she cries. This is a waste of energy. Just pick her up. Try different approaches to comforting her until you hit on one that works. Being there with some kind of a response is more important than getting the right one on the first try. Babies cry for a lot of reasons. Hunger is one, boredom is another, being too hot or too cold is a third. Some babies hate being in a wet diaper. Others don't seem to notice.

Most often, the answer to your baby's cry is you—a person, not a clean diaper, not a fancy mobile, not a cradle or a baby swing. There is so much equipment available for holding babies that we forget that the most natural, emotionally healthful place for an infant to be is in her mother's arms. Most babies don't like to be put down for very long. If holding your baby much of the time keeps her from crying, then that's what you should do. (The subject of "babywearing" is coming up soon.)

This sounds simple, but new mothers often worry about whether jumping every time the baby cries is the right thing to do. You start to feel as if the baby is controlling you, and you wonder if this sets a bad pattern for the months and years to follow. Aren't you rewarding the baby for crying if you respond even when she's only bored or lonely? The answer is no. Remember, a baby's cry is her language, and you want to communicate with her. When you respond to her cries, you are rewarding her for trying to talk to you, trying to connect and find comfort when she's feeling out of sorts. You want her to reach out for human contact. Think how important it is to have this ability, both as a child and as an adult. With time, your baby will find ways other than crying to get your attention, and she'll do it faster if you reward her efforts to communicate.

So when your baby is crying, don't think that you have to make her stop just for the sake of ending the noise. Try to discover the reason for the cry, and you will both be on your way to healthy mother-and-child commu-nication. And you can feel good about finding what works when your baby cries.

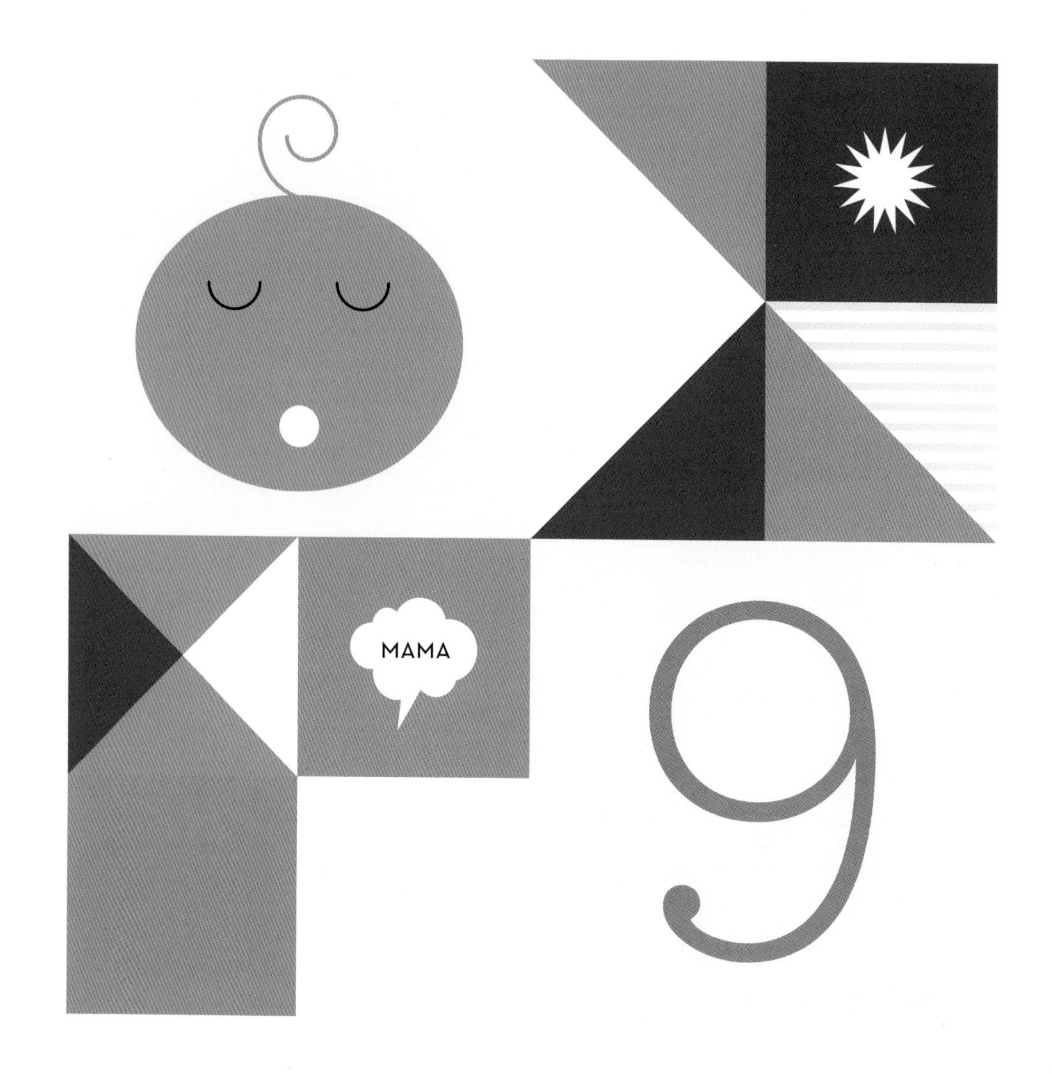
MAMA
9

Your Baby Needs You Close by Day

Your baby is going to want to be in your arms as much as he can. He has his reasons—good ones. You may have reasons for wanting to put him down—you need your hands free or maybe your arms are ready to give out. Is a conflict brewing here?

Try "babywearing," a time-tested, multicultural, practical, and fun solution to the question "How will I ever get anything done?" Wearing the baby, using a sling or other carrier, is an old, old custom, practiced by women around the world. I'm not talking here about using the carrier only for walks or trips to the park or grocery store. Use it all the time, at home as well as away. Carry your baby for several hours each day, and you'll be very pleased with the results. One study showed that babies who were carried this way cried 43 percent less than others. Most mothers don't need a study to convince them that carrying the baby keeps him happy.

A carried baby is a peaceful baby. He's up where things are happening, where he can hear Mom's voice, feel her motion. Mother's closeness helps him to organize his behavior. He fusses less and spends more time quiet and alert, learning about the world. He's usually a joy to be with, and this makes his parents want to carry him even more.

Meanwhile, you are free to go about your routine. You can putter around in the kitchen, vacuum, play with the baby's siblings, or take a long hike in the woods. Wearing your baby makes it easy to go places. You can squeeze between the racks at crowded stores in the mall, and you don't have to go looking for ramps and elevators, as you would if you were pushing a

A carried baby is a peaceful baby.

stroller. And you won't find yourself awkwardly trying to push an empty stroller while carrying the cranky baby who refuses to ride in it.

Babywearing makes it possible to take your baby to places where infants don't usually go. A baby who is carried in a sling much of the time learns to feel content there, whatever the larger surroundings. I've found that my babies have been happy and content in the baby sling in all kinds of situations—church services, medical meetings, parties, airplane trips, even live television appearances. I've been able to do things and go places that wouldn't have been possible otherwise. Babywearing has kept me from feeling tied down when I have a baby who is unhappy being away from me.

I have found that a sling-type carrier works the best. It's easy to put on; it slips over your head, and the baby slips right in. With practice you can put it on without setting the baby down. You can adjust it easily with the baby inside, and you can take it off to lay a sleeping baby down without awakening him. The model most commonly sold in stores is padded at the shoulder for the mother's comfort and along the edges for the baby's comfort. You can wear a sling over or under a jacket or sweater. Best of all, it's the only kind of carrier you'll need to buy: You can use it with a newborn, an older baby, and on up through toddlerhood. Your baby can lie cradled inside or snuggled against your chest, sit facing forward kangaroo-style, or straddle your hip. You can even breastfeed discreetly with the baby in the sling, while you're sitting down or strolling along. There are many subtle variations on the basic positions, so you and your baby can figure out what works for you at each developmental stage.

Front-pack carriers suit newborns and sleeping babies, but a baby of three or four months wants to look around, and he can't do that very well while squashed against your chest, where most front-packs require him to be. Since front-packs also can put quite a strain on the mother's back and are not safe around stoves, families who start off with these carriers often discontinue using them after a few months. Back-pack carriers, the ones with aluminum frames, can't be used until a baby is about three months old, and a major disadvantage is that you can't see the baby. (You may get your hair pulled, too.) Backpacks do keep the baby out of the way while you're slicing onions, but most women find that they are more comfortable with a sling, which puts much of the baby's weight directly on the mother's hip, rather than pulling down on her shoulders. And with practice you can even sling your baby around to your back when you need to slice onions.

Using a sling—or any type of baby carrier—does take some practice. You need time to get the hang of it and to learn to trust the sling to keep your baby safe. Your baby also may take a few days getting used to being carried this way, so don't give up if the baby fusses the first few times you try wearing him. Babywearing is good for both of you, so gently teach your baby to appreciate it. One tip for getting started: As soon as you get the baby into the sling, start moving; walk, jiggle, pat his bottom to help him settle into this new feeling. Some babies prefer to be more upright in the sling. Experiment with new positions as your baby's ability to support his head and neck improve.

Wearing your baby is especially helpful in the late afternoon, when there may be a great deal of commotion in the household, with older kids coming and going and a meal to prepare. You can also wear a baby down to sleep, even one who is very wound up and determined to stay awake. Just put the baby in the sling and start walking. Take a stroll outside or around the house, go put in a load of laundry, or sort your junk mail while standing and swaying at the kitchen table. Or try breastfeeding the baby in the sling while you're moving gently. He may be asleep in no time.

Babywearing will help you connect with your baby at times when you might not be feeling very motherly. If you're having

Over a period of many years, I have watched hundreds of "sling babies" and their mothers parade through my pediatric office.

There is a beautiful difference about these babies and their mothers. The babies seem content; they cry less; they enjoy eye contact because they are used to it, and they become sociable children because they have been so intimately involved in the world of the mothers who carried them. Some mothers in our pediatric practice even wear their babies on the job—we call it work-and-wear. This age-old custom of babywearing is finally catching on in Western culture, and I believe we will see a whole crop of more intimately attached parents and babies as a result. One of my fondest memories as a father is wearing our babies in a sling around the house, shopping, and around the park. Our children may never remember those precious moments in the baby sling, but I shall never forget them.

—Bill

a down day, keeping your baby close to you will help stimulate good feelings. If your baby is having a day when he is being very demanding (maybe because of a growth spurt, a cold coming on, teething, or just the stress of normal development), wearing him will make it much easier for you to meet his needs. If you're just not sure what's going on with him, put him in the baby sling. You'll save yourself the stress of making the should-I-pick-him-up-or-not decision 30 or 40 times a day. Day in and day out, babywearing will make you more sensitive to your baby's cues and more confident as a mother.

You may run into people who insist that you're spoiling your baby by carrying him all the time, or that he'll never learn to crawl if you don't leave him on the floor. Remember, these people have no biological connection to your baby. Nor do they have your minute-by-minute expertise in interpreting his cues. Carrying babies doesn't spoil them. It turns them into delightful little human beings, who want to be carried some more because they feel good that way. Eventually, your baby will want some floor time, to kick his feet and explore the concept of locomotion. He'll let you know, and because you've carried him so much, you'll have little trouble figuring out when he wants down.

So give babywearing a try. Baby slings come in a variety of prints and patterns. Choose one that coordinates well with your wardrobe, and your parenting choices become a fashion statement as well. Baby slings can be bought at almost any baby store and in baby sections of department stores. For information on where to buy a popular model, the Balboa Baby, in your area or to order online, visit www.BalboaBaby.com.

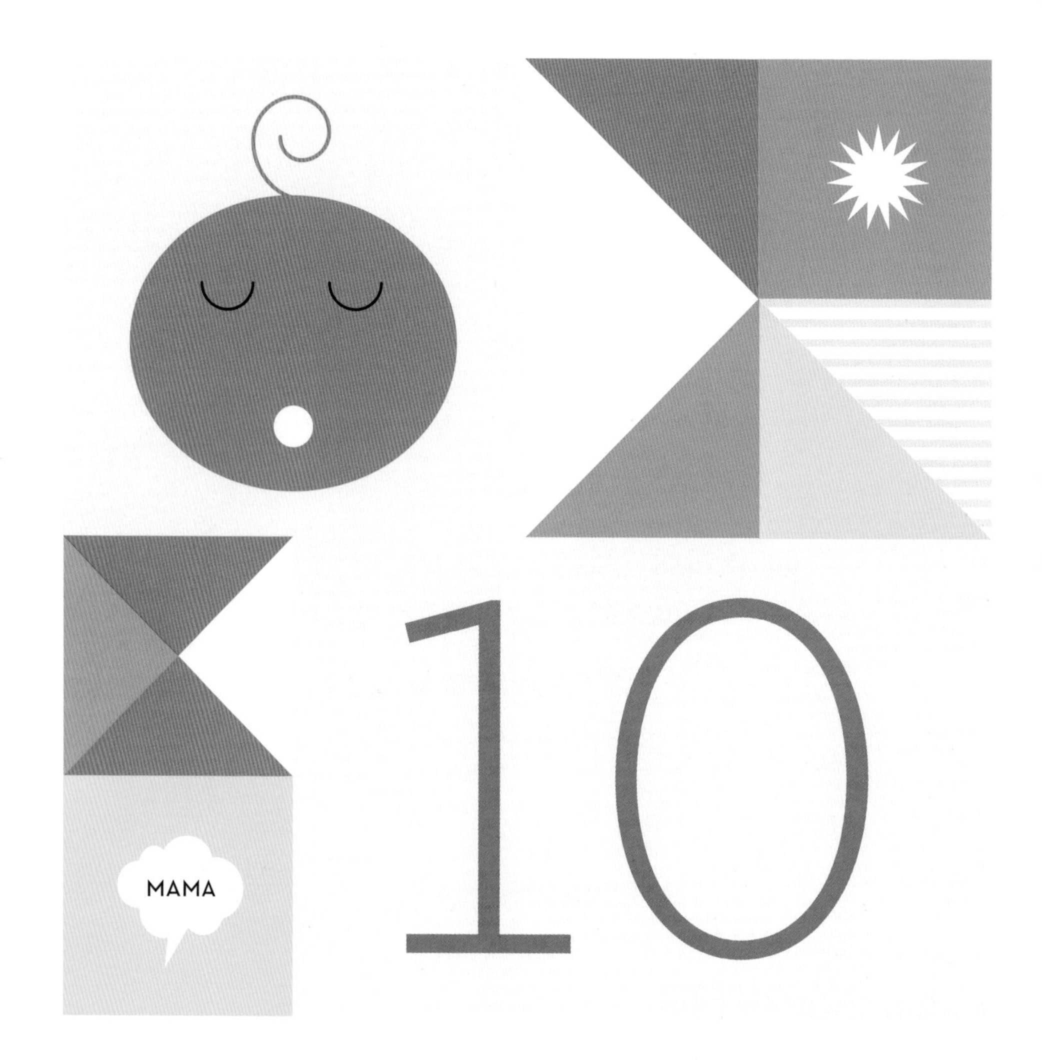
MAMA
10

Your Baby Needs You Close by Night

A baby who is close to her mother all day is going to want to continue the good feelings into the nighttime. The big, lonely crib or even the snug, cozy bassinet is not going to provide these for her. She craves the back-to-the-womb feeling of being close to Mom, so she wants warmth, that certain smell, the feeling of a soft body gently breathing near her.

You could invest in tapes of womb sounds, a crib that jiggles babies to sleep automatically, and a hammock that snuggles them, but if your baby is like most babies, she would still clamor for you. She needs you all the more when she is tired or when she awakens frightened and hungry in the middle of the night.

Fortunately, there's another age-old, multicultural, practical, and pleasurable custom that will take care of these needs and allow you to get some sleep as well. We call it sharing sleep. Actually, in most cultures it's not called anything because people just assume that a baby sleeps with her mother. The practice of sharing sleep is as old as the human race, and it persists because it works so well. Even in our "advanced" culture, many parents share sleep with their children at one time or another. Unfortunately, they've had so many experts over the years tell them that they shouldn't do this that they're often afraid to admit that they do.

Sharing sleep means keeping your baby close to you at night so that you can meet her nighttime needs. When your baby sleeps next to you, it's easy to breastfeed at night. As your baby wakens and starts squirming around in search of the nipple, you wake up, too, pull her in close to you, get her started at the breast, and then drift back to sleep. Your baby doesn't have

Sharing sleep means keeping your baby close to you at night so that you can meet her nighttime needs.

to cry, and you don't have to get out of bed or even wake up completely.

Sharing sleep also meets your baby's nighttime need for closeness. She'll actually sleep better with her mother next to her than she will by herself. A baby's cycles of light and deep sleep are shorter than an adult's. During the time the baby is moving from one kind of sleep to another, she is more likely to awaken. Because babies have a lot of these transition periods every night, they have many opportunities for night-waking. However, if your warm, familiar body is close by, your baby is able to handle these transitions more easily. Your sleeping presence keeps her calm, and she is more likely to move on to the next sleep stage without crying. Your presence may also prevent her from sleeping too deeply, which could make her vulnerable to the arousal problems researchers associate with Sudden Infant Death Syndrome (SIDS).

A lot of neat things happen when you share sleep with your baby. First of all, the two of you get your sleep cycles synchronized. So you tend to be in light sleep when the baby wakes for feedings, and because you haven't been dragged out of a deep sleep, you feel more rested in the morning. You also get to share some very special times with your baby. You can reach out and touch her as you're falling asleep. You can watch her little sleep grins and share these funny expressions with your partner. You can wake up every morning with a cheerful baby and feel blessed and amazed all over again that she is so beautiful and so special.

Does taking your baby into your bed every night sound radical to you? I can understand this. It took me four babies to figure out that I didn't have to sit up for night feedings and then

---

Here are some practical tips for sharing sleep safely:

Push your bed flush against the wall or use a guardrail, and fill in any gaps with a tightly rolled baby blanket. Place your baby between her mother and the wall or rail. Mothers are physically and mentally aware of their babies even while sleeping, but fathers do not have the same level of awareness. Use a big bed with plenty of room for everyone, or use an Arm's Reach Bedside Co-Sleeper, a crib-like bassinet that attaches safely and securely to the parents' bed (see www.armsreach.com). Do not sleep with your baby on a couch; she may get wedged between your body and the couch cushions. Don't sleep with your baby if you are under the influence of alcohol or any drug that diminishes your awareness of your baby.

No matter where your baby sleeps, avoid putting her to sleep on a squishy surface, such as a wavy waterbed or a beanbag chair. And put her to sleep on her back; this decreases the risk of Sudden Infant Death Syndrome (SIDS).

—Bill

try to ease a sleeping baby back into a crib, so I can appreciate the shift in thinking necessary to see sleep sharing as a simple, natural part of parenting.

Consider again that you and your baby are not quite separate people yet. You are still linked together mentally and emotionally as well as biologically through breastfeeding. Putting your baby to sleep in the nursery down the hall puts a lot of stress on this connection. Both you and your baby feel anxious away from each other. You lie awake listening for the baby, and the baby feels scared and angry when she awakens alone.

At the same time, however, there are social pressures at work on you. We live in a culture that prizes independence, and modern parents are told to teach their babies to sleep on their own, to be happy with substitute caregivers, and even to comfort themselves when they cry. But this is not how true independence develops. Before a baby can be independent she must soak up all the positive feelings about herself that come from a close connection to her mother (and her father, too). Experiencing the interdependence of the mother-baby bond is the best way for a baby to grow toward independence. Being able to depend on her mother teaches the baby eventually to trust herself, and this self-trust is the foundation of independent living.

Sleep sharing fits in nicely with today's busy lifestyles, especially when both parents are employed. It allows parents to reconnect with the baby at night, making up for the time they didn't have close to the baby during the day. We have observed that babies who sleep with their parents develop a healthy attitude about sleep—that sleep, for them, is a pleasant state to enter and a secure state to remain in. I am certain that if we took a poll and asked babies where they wanted to sleep, their overwhelming response would be "With my parents, of course!" Isn't that the natural place to be? I believe that science will soon prove what intuitive parents have long known, that something good and healthful occurs between parents and baby when they share sleep.

—Bill

You may feel that you need to get away from your baby at night in order to take a break from being a mother. Or you might think that you just won't sleep well with your baby next to you. These are certainly legitimate feelings, and you shouldn't force yourself to persist with sharing sleep out of a sense of grim duty. You can be responsive to a baby's nighttime needs in other ways, too. But it wouldn't hurt to give sleep sharing a try for a week or more. It can really help you relax into motherhood.

The best place for a baby to sleep, generally, is between her mother and the wall or a guardrail. Some fathers are not as aware of a tiny baby's whereabouts as mothers tend to be. And although some dads like their babies in the middle, putting your baby between you and the edge of the bed gives you and your husband an opportunity to be close and avoids sending the message that the baby has come between you. Sleep sharing doesn't have to interfere with your cuddle time. As for lovemaking, there are other places in the house where you can relax and enjoy each other (a couch, living room carpet, spare bedroom, foam mattresses on the bedroom floor, or even just the other half of the bed if the baby is sound asleep and you can be really quiet). Or you can put the baby in the crib for the first part of the night and bring her into your bed when you're ready to go to sleep.

Sleep sharing won't teach your baby to sleep through the night at an early age, and it won't teach her to find her thumb and comfort herself back to sleep. There are sleep "experts" out there who will warn you that letting your baby fall asleep at the breast and offering your presence and some nursing when she awakens will create poor sleep habits; the baby will depend on you for help in getting to sleep and will even think that you don't trust her to fall asleep on her own.

They're partly right. Yes, having you there when she goes to sleep will become a habit, a very nice one that may continue into the years of bedtime stories, good-night prayers, and special tuck-in rituals. Sharing sleep will help your child grow up with a good attitude toward sleep, and this is far more important in the prevention of later sleep problems than how long it takes for a child to learn to fall asleep on her own. When your baby sleeps with you, you are actually teaching her how to enjoy sleep. What a restful lesson to learn!

You can put the baby in the crib for the first part of the night and bring her into your bed when you're ready to go to sleep.

MAMA
11

Beware the Self-Soothing Baby

The fifties had the Dr. Spock babies, the sixties and seventies the all-natural babies, and the eighties the stimulated superbabies. Today's babies are the self-soothing babies, the newest in a long line of baby-rearing fads.

The self-soothing baby is the one who finds his fingers and sucks on them instead of crying out for Mom. He puts himself back to sleep when he awakens in the middle of the night, without needing a feeding and with a minimum of fuss. He is content to hang out on the fringes of mother's life, watching, leaving her free to do all of the important things a 21st-century woman's life is full of. He's a very convenient fellow to have around.

By now, you may be asking: "What's wrong with self-soothing?" and/or "Why isn't my baby like that?"

Most babies are not self-soothers when they are born. They are born instead with the ability and the drive to summon help. If they could not do this, they would not be able to command the level of parenting they need to get their needs met. If a newborn baby could consistently chew on his fist to quiet himself down, how would his mother know when to feed him? How would he get the stimulation he needs from being picked up and carried around on his mother's shoulder? A very sensitive mother who is well attuned to the needs of infants will do these things whether her baby requests them or not (and if you have a very easygoing baby you should take the lead and pay attention to him even though he may not cry or fuss very much). A woman who is just learning to be a mother or who is preoccupied with other matters might not give her baby all the attention he needs to develop to his highest potential.

There's nothing wrong with a baby learning to soothe himself as he grows older. Teaching your baby to be able to restore his inner feelings of rightness on his own is one of your goals as a parent. There's a good way to do this and a way that has potential for harm.

The good way starts with not expecting your baby to take care of his own needs, because you understand that he is really not ready to do this yet. Instead, you concentrate on responding to your baby's cries for help and teaching him what it is like to feel right inside, to feel content. He also learns to trust you, his caregiving world, and this, too, helps him know that he is entitled to have good feelings. Eventually you find that you can slightly lengthen the time it takes you to respond when your baby is fussing without having him go all to pieces. Some of these times he may actually solve his problems on his own without your coming at all. He will have become so accustomed to the pattern of comfort following distress that he will sometimes be able to restore his good mood on his own.

I can't tell you at what age this will begin to happen for your baby—it depends on your baby's temperament and what is going on in your lives. But it will happen, very gradually, if you let it. Of course, if you hear those preliminary fussing noises begin to escalate into a cry, you should step in and help your baby pull himself back together.

Letting your baby cry it out might also eventually teach him to soothe himself, but this road to having a self-soothing baby has its dangers. The baby learns to soothe himself because he discovers he has no other choice—no one will help him. He stops crying out of despair, not because he has learned to recover good feelings on his own. His trust in his parents is shaken, and he decides he must tough it out on his own in a hard world. From this treatment he emerges harboring negative feelings that may contribute to a poor sense of self-worth in the years to come.

Letting a baby cry it out is tough on mothers as well. If you try it, it will probably feel wrong to you. The urge to help your baby when he cries is a strong one, and a mother's heart does not harden easily when it comes to her baby's happiness. But many books out today suggest some form of crying it out as the answer to all the demands an infant places on his busy parents. This advice, which should have gone out with wringer washers and starched shirt collars, is back in full force. Recognize it when you see it as advice that is parent-centered—that is, geared toward a father and mother's convenience. It is not really in your baby's interest.

There are all kinds of mother substitutes that also promise to calm your baby in your place—swings, pacifiers, audio tapes, bouncing seats, and more. These have their place, filling in for mother when she is ready to give out, but think of them as your emergency backup crew, not the ordinary day- and night-shift workers. In years gone by a new mother was not expected to take care of a baby on her own all day long. She had an extended family who shared the daily baby care. Though times have changed, babies still need human arms whenever possible. When your baby grows into a child and eventually into an adult, you don't want him to turn to things for comfort when he is feeling distressed. You want him to be able to rely on his own inner resources and the people who love him.

I wonder if those who advise mothers to let their babies cry it out were themselves as infants victims of self-soothing advice; perhaps they have carried this insensitivity into their own parenting.

A baby's cry is a baby's language. It is designed for the survival of the baby and the development of the mother. Advising a mother to let her baby cry goes against both common sense and what we know of maternal biology. When a baby cries, a mother responds with an overwhelming physiological urge to pick up and comfort her baby. Studies have even shown that the mother's blood flow to her breasts increases in response to her baby's cries. These biological responses occur for a reason. Listen to them. It's easy for someone else to advise a mother to let her baby cry, because that person is not biologically wired to the baby. I advise a mother never to go against what her biology tells her; otherwise the result will be insensitivity and a developing distance between mother and baby.

—Bill

MAMA
12

You Really Do Have Intuition

You don't have to be a mother of eight children to have intuition. All you have to do is spend a lot of time with your baby.

The more interaction you have with your baby, the better developed your intuition about her will be.

A mother's intuition is nothing more than quick and ready insight into her children's behavior. It isn't ESP; it isn't some strange psychic resonance between mother and child. Your intuition is based on an accumulation of observations about your baby, little bits and pieces of information that are stored in your brain and can be used to form reasonable hypotheses about what your baby is thinking or how she will react. When your baby scowls or laughs, your brain scans back through all these "bytes" of information and uses them to interpret her behavior. This process takes a lot longer to read about than it does to happen. You just feel you know what is going on with your baby.

Intuitive knowledge of your baby can be a very valuable thing to have. It tips you off when your baby isn't feeling well. Even before you get out the thermometer, you know she is sick. You can sense when her fussiness is from a busy day and when it is caused by discomfort from teething or an ear infection. Intuition tells you when it's time for you and the baby to leave the party and go to a quiet room to nurse. It tells you why your baby is crying and what makes her feel safe and secure.

You acquire the information on which intuition is based during everyday living. The more interaction you have with your baby, the better developed your intuition about her will be.

A theory based on experiments with several hundred subjects is more reliable than one based on a study of only 40 or 50 cases. Each time your baby gives a cue and you respond, you are building a store of knowledge that will help you to respond even better the next time.

In many ways, saying that you have mother's intuition is just another way of saying that you have learned a great deal about your baby. Your baby wakes howling furiously, and you respond by offering the breast—which worked the last time you heard her howl. But the baby turns away and continues to cry, and you notice a new intensity in the cry. Maybe something is hurting her. It's not the pain of a hungry tummy, because she didn't want to nurse. So you check her sleeper and discover a tiny thread wrapped tightly around two of her toes. Ouch! This incident both uses and builds your intuition. You've used your intuition to know that this cry requires action from you, and you've also added the shrieking sound of a pain cry to your intuition's memory bank for future reference.

Mother's intuition is grounded in information collected by all the senses. How your baby's body feels, her smell, her noises, her cuddly times, her active times all help you to know her better. This is why it is so helpful to your mothering if you keep your baby against your body. You can put all of your mind—not just the thinking part—to work on the job of getting to know your child.

What if you feel that you don't have any intuition? Don't worry about it. Just focus on your baby. Keep experimenting with responses to her cues until you find ones that work. Be flexible, and really observe. Try to let go of preconceptions you may have brought to parenting—ideas like "Babies sleep all the time" or "Scheduled feedings are best." Your baby may be trying to teach you something quite different, and, if you are willing to learn, both of you will benefit. As you discover all the things your baby is trying to tell you and all the ways you can communicate your love back to her, a wonderful trust will grow up between you. Call it harmony, call it mutual giving, call it intuitive mothering—it will feel right to you and to your baby. You'll just know it.

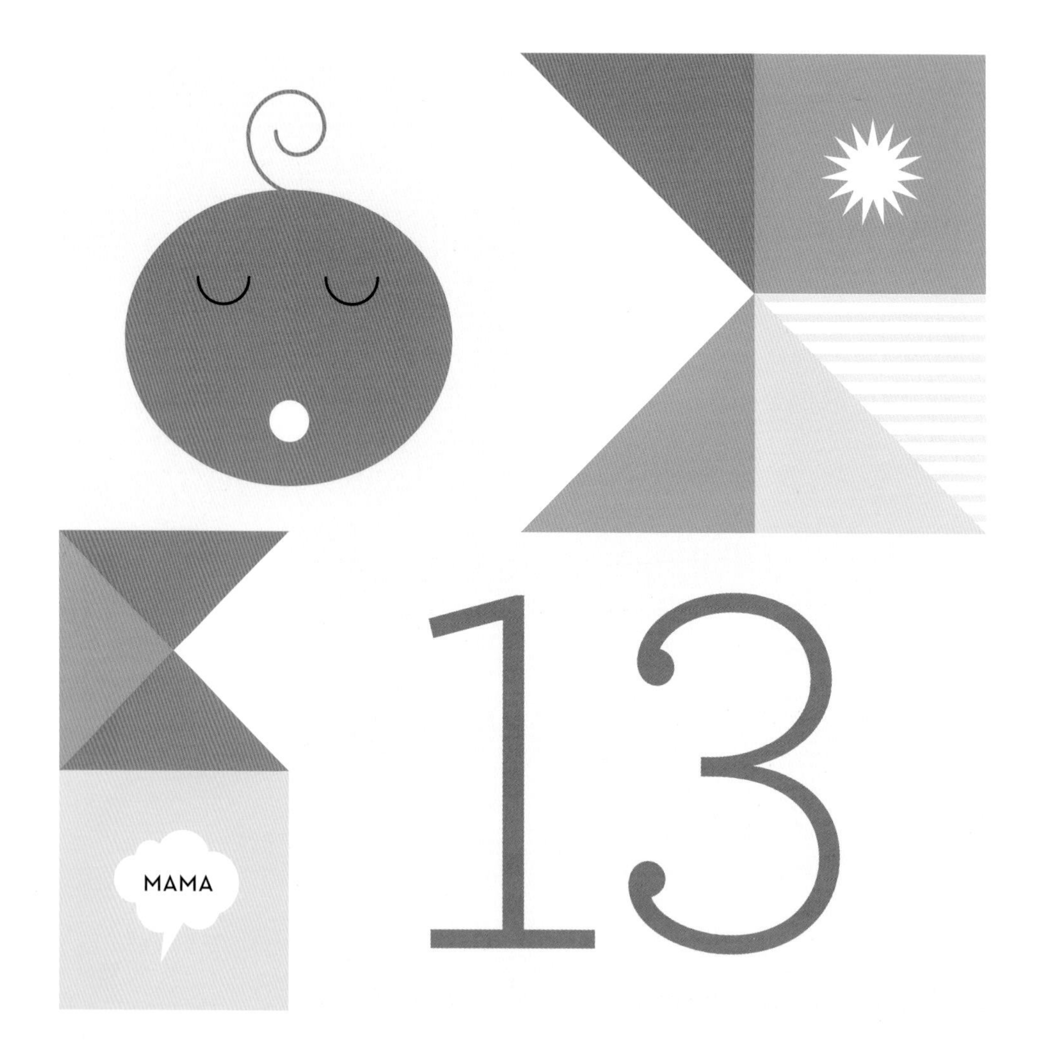
MAMA
13

Things Will Never Be "Normal" Again

Holidays are nice, vacations are fun, special events add spark to everyday life, but there's always something comforting about getting back to normal. Variety may be the spice of life, but daily routines help us feel secure and in control.

When will things get back to normal after you have a new baby? I guess that depends on what you mean by "normal." If you mean, "When will there be some kind of established routine to our lives?", "When will I be able to count on taking a shower every day?", "When will I not feel so new at this?", the answer is "Soon." Exactly when will vary with the temperament of your baby, your lifestyle, and your ability to remain flexible. If by "normal" you mean, "When will I feel as I did before the baby came?", "When will life be simpler?", "When will my baby stop making so many demands on me?", brace yourself, because the answer is "Never." Things will never be this kind of normal again.

Life changes profoundly when you have a child, to a degree that's hard to anticipate before he's born. You're no longer the person you were before you had a baby. You don't think of yourself or your husband first any more, you think of the baby. Everything is more complicated, from making love to making dinner, and there's no getting away from it. This is what's normal now.

You will settle into this new way of life. After a month or two you'll emerge from your postpartum haze and once again notice the world around you. You'll get used to your baby's

The hallmark of babyhood is change.

constant presence, and you'll be better able to anticipate his needs. You'll understand yourself as a mother better, and you'll feel more sure of yourself.

Nevertheless, the hallmark of babyhood is change. As soon as you get one stage figured out, you're on to the next one. One day holding is all it takes to comfort your baby; two weeks later his fussing sounds mean that he needs a walk around the house because he's bored. Next month he'll be fussing about something else, wanting to be put down on the floor or carried facing forward. This rapid progress through developmental stages is fun to witness, but it can leave you a little off balance—and looking for a more stable version of normality.

Longing for things to get back to normal can also mean wanting your body back the way it was. Nine months of pregnancy followed by breastfeeding leaves some women feeling at odds with their physical selves. Leaking milk, clothes that don't fit, and, if your baby is sensitive to foods you eat (this sort of sensitivity is not all that common, but does sometimes occur), a restricted diet can grow tiresome. Sharing your body with your baby can become a symbol of just how much control you've lost over your moment-to-moment existence.

There are ways to cope when you yearn for normality—things to do that stop short of weaning your baby, returning to work ahead of schedule, or signing up for a cruise to the Greek islands. One, or a combination of several, may work for you.

First is the pamper-yourself approach. This recognizes that new mothers deserve a break. Think of the first few months postpartum as a prolonged honeymoon with your baby, and indulge yourself. Take a nap when the baby sleeps. Buy your favorite out-of-season fresh fruit at the store, or order a carry-out dinner from a favorite restaurant. Take long baths with your baby. Read the latest page-turning paperback while you nurse. Let the baby nurse the morning away in bed with you while you sleep late.

Another strategy is to pick out one or two things in your life and work on getting those under control. The satisfaction of cleaning out the kitchen junk drawer and getting it thoroughly organized can make you forget that the rest of the house is a mess. Shopping for one nice outfit that fits and flatters and is easy to nurse in can help you cope with the nothing-to-wear blues. If predictability is important to you, resolve to make the bed or write a letter to someone every day, or get out for a daily walk. Set yourself up for success by choosing tasks that don't take too long, can be done in stages days apart, or can be done easily with the baby in tow. Accomplishing one or two small things like this every few days takes the bite out of the feeling that you can never get anything done. Pat yourself heartily on the back every time you even attempt a small project.

A third approach is remembering that the time when your baby is small is very short in the overall scheme of things. Babies grow up all too quickly. When you're sending this child off to college, on his first date, or even just to kindergarten, you'll want to have a storehouse of lovely memories to look back on as you dab at your eyes with a tissue. Life may seem a lot more normal at that point, but you'll be thinking of these baby days nostalgically. One way to make them memorable is to keep your mind and emotions on your life here and now. Enjoy the present with your baby, even if it seems a far cry from "normal."

MAMA
14

Playtime Is All the Time

You don't have to make a big project out of playing with your baby. Playtime is all the time. Having fun is naturally part of baby care. The secret is to relax enough to realize you are having fun.

You are your baby's very best and most educational toy. In the first several months, almost everything she learns comes from you. She discovers herself and much about the world by observing and interacting with the person who is most important to her, her mother. The shelves at the toy store may be loaded with enticing gadgets that promise to build a better, smarter baby, but none of them can compare with the ever-changing, always interesting face of a parent.

You are both your baby's window to the world and a mirror that reflects her back to herself. You'll want to keep those surfaces bright and clean. If you feel harried and tense, at odds with the world and all the people in it, your baby gets that view, too. If you go through the day with your lips pursed in anger, your baby takes that in as an image of herself. She will pick up on your tension and internalize the emotions behind your scowl.

There will be days and times when your glass is going to be clouded, and that's okay. Babies can take the occasional bad day along with the good, but, for the most part, you want to show your baby a cheerful, happy image of herself and her surroundings. (If for you the bad days are far outnumbering the good ones, this is a sign that you should seek help in changing your life and outlook.) On the glum days, when baby care or being stuck at home in midwinter is getting you down, taking a few minutes to play with your baby can help to polish your glass. Putting on a happy face can transform your inner mood, especially when you see your baby respond to attention.

You don't have to plan an elaborate play session with your baby. You can have fun when you're changing diapers. Smile and make silly sounds to keep the baby from wiggling. Put on some music and sing and dance with your baby while you wear her around the house (this can make cleaning a little more tolerable). Talk to her while you make your way around the supermarket. See that she has interesting things to look at—the dining room chandelier while you're eating dinner, a mobile or two hung where she will notice as you pass by, the view through a window that you gaze out of together. Help her learn to enjoy a bath by taking her into the tub with you. (To get in safely, put the baby in a towel-lined baby seat right next to the tub, get in yourself, sit down, and lean over the side to pick up the baby. To get out, lean over and put the baby in the seat, wrap the towel around her, and get out yourself. Or get Dad to help.) Your baby needs you to let go of some of that seriousness that comes with being a responsible parent. Whether it's Bach or Beatles, the mall or a museum, share the everyday things you enjoy with your baby.

You will also want to take some special time out each day to concentrate on your baby and everything she can do. Keep her on your lap at first, and play with her on the floor as she gets bigger. Choose a time when she's in a good mood, quiet and alert. Hold her so that you can look each other in the face, and talk to her in a gentle voice, using her name. Show her a few simple toys, preferably ones that make noise. Try to get her eyes to follow. She can track moving objects with her eyes a bit even as a newborn. You might even see her imitate your facial expressions. As she gets older, your conversations will grow more animated; she'll giggle and coo. She'll be able to swipe at rattles and eventually grab them. Lying on her tummy on the floor, she'll lift her head to look at you. One day she'll surprise you (and probably herself) by rolling onto her back.

Basic knowledge of infant development will help you to play games appropriate for your baby's age and even to challenge her to move on to the next stage. You don't have to be an expert, but consulting some kind of guide will help you recognize new skills as they emerge and know what to expect next (see Resources, page 203, for some suggestions on books to read). Keeping a journal of your playtime with your baby is a great way to record her individual development and preserve for posterity all the wonderful things you discover together.

Basic knowledge of infant development will help you to play games appropriate for your baby's age and even to challenge her to move on to the next stage.

As you play with your baby, be sensitive to her reactions. Some babies like things loud and boisterous; others are quieter and more reserved. Honor your baby's unique personality by respecting her choices in play. She'll learn much more if you follow her cues rather than making her follow yours or the book's. Playtime involves a lot of give and take. This is a time to really observe your baby and figure out what she likes.

Respect your baby's stop signals. Babies need to take frequent breaks from stimulation. Your baby will look away from you when she needs a short break. Wait for her to return her focus to your face. It's okay to woo a baby back gently, but be careful not to overwhelm her or she may get so wound up that she explodes into crying.

Infant massage is a relaxing way to play with a baby, especially a young one who hasn't yet developed a lot of other ways to play. You can learn infant massage from a book (Vimala Schneider McClure's *Infant Massage: A Handbook for Loving Parents* has excellent photographs), from DVDs, or from a class with a certified infant-massage instructor (see Resources, page 202). Some babies like morning massages; some find massage helpful just before the late-afternoon fussy hour begins. Besides having great play value, massage promotes growth in babies, improves their digestion, calms their nerves, and helps them learn to appreciate their bodies. Massaging your infant will also relax you, help you feel more motherly, and build your intuition. As you watch your baby relax and feel good all over, you'll gain a new appreciation of her many moods and become more confident handling her. I enjoyed the way massage helped me memorize every square inch of my babies' delightful little bodies. Infant massage is great for dads to learn, too; it gives them a sense of intimacy with the baby that they might not otherwise find.

You and your baby will find many special ways to enjoy each other. You'll share your own silly "ga-ga" language. You'll make faces and grin at each other. You may invent cute names for her like "Pumpkin" or "Itty Bitty Ba." Daily rituals will evolve that both of you will treasure. You may be the only one who remembers them five or ten years from now, but your child will enjoy hearing about them. "Tell me about when I was a baby," she'll say, as she cuddles up to you. You'll be happy to oblige, remembering how the love you share was nurtured by these first play sessions.

MAMA
15

You Can Get the Baby's Father Involved

A dad who can calm a fussy baby, entertain a bored baby, and sometimes put a tired baby to sleep is a blessing to both mother and child.

Father involvement works best if it starts early—if the two of you learn together about caring for your baby. This is not as easy as it sounds. You, the mother, have a biological connection to your baby that began in pregnancy and continues in breastfeeding. When the baby is upset, you take it a lot more personally than Dad does. Your milk leaks, you hurry to pick up the baby, your face shows concern, the comforting words come out of your mouth more or less automatically (depending perhaps on how stressed out you are). Even if your plans for the future include returning to work, you're probably taking a longer parental leave than your husband is, and both of you probably assume that Mom will be the baby's primary caregiver for at least the first few months.

Add to all this the fact that the new father's store of baby-care experience is probably even smaller than yours, and you have a man who may have a lot of doubts about his baby-tending qualifications. Even though warm and cuddly pictures of dads and babies are starting to appear in magazine advertisements for soap and blue jeans, the stereotype persists of the bumbling male who barely knows which end of the baby is which. A father may long for a close relationship with his baby, but he may not know how to achieve it.

You must stand back and let your partner find his own way. His style of comforting and playing with your baby will not be the same as yours, and the temptation to swoop in and take over will be great. But if you're always there to rescue the baby from Dad, how will Dad ever learn, much less acquire any confidence? If the baby is fussing in Dad's arms, keep your distance—let the two of them work things out. If the baby is becoming more upset and Dad is growing more frustrated, you will have to step in. Do this in a way that doesn't cast aspersions on your husband's parenting skills—"Maybe he's hungry; I'll see if he wants to nurse."

Give your partner opportunities to practice his baby-care skills. After breastfeeding the baby, hand him off to Dad and go take a long shower or soak in the tub. Send the two of them out on a walk around the block. Take time for yourself every day (you need it!) while Dad takes care of the baby.

Some babies are at times unwilling to hang out with Dad. Let your partner know that he should not take this personally or make himself scarce; the baby likes him nearby, just not too nearby. There will be times when the baby will welcome Dad's fresh set of arms, and you'll wonder what your partner did to calm your infant. Dad will feel like a hero, and you'll appreciate him to no end.

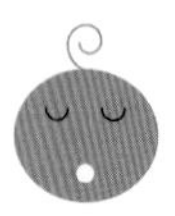

Dad can take over baths, burping, or walking the baby when he needs to settle down.

Breastfeeding sometimes appears to stand in the way of a father's developing a close relationship with his baby. Because you do all the feeding, the most time-consuming part of baby care, Dad may feel as if there's nothing important left for him to do. He may want to join in by giving the baby a bottle. Instead of assenting, ask for help with other tasks. Dad can take over baths, burping, or walking the baby when he needs to settle down. Most fathers want to be left out of baby care at night, but if your mate craves involvement, he can share the work in the wee hours by taking over nighttime diapering and burping. Even holding and breathing on a sleeping baby who might wake up if placed on a cold crib mattress can be a special role for a father.

The intimacy of the breastfeeding relationship may make a father feel jealous if he didn't get enough mothering when he was little. If this is a sensitive area for your husband, he will need to suppress his feelings to avoid adding stress to your life. A jealous Dad can cause a new mother to feel guilty about her devotion to her baby and to doubt her maternal intuition and responsiveness. If this is happening in your family, talk the matter over with someone who can help you assess the situation. Your childbirth educator or your birth attendant might be a good person to talk with. Then, maybe all you will need to do is talk things over honestly and caringly with your mate. Just knowing you understand his feelings may be healing for him. If not, he may need professional counseling to help him feel comfortable in his new role. Becoming a parent—a mother or a father—is, after all, one of life's major adjustments.

Share what you learn about your baby with your husband. Give helpful information, perhaps from the baby's viewpoint—for example, "He likes to be up on your shoulder" or "He's had a hard day, lots of new experiences." This will get a better response than "Don't hold him like that" or "No, don't take him to Kmart!" New fathers are sensitive, just like new mothers. Nagging and bossing leave them feeling inadequate and shut out.

Talk with your husband about a parenting philosophy the two of you can share. Dads are not always eager readers of child-care books and magazines. They often depend on their wives to tell them what they most need to know. Be sure your husband understands how important it is to be responsive to your baby's cues. This will help him understand why you jump whenever the baby cries. It will also motivate him to pay more attention to the baby's signals. If Dad understands that you are laying the foundation for your child's sense of self and trust, he will be more tolerant of interrupted conversations, late dinners, and night-waking episodes.

In these first weeks postpartum, you need your partner to take care of you as well as to help with baby care. He can't do this unless you tell him specifically what you need. Men are no better at reading minds than women are (they may not even be as good). Your husband may be totally mystified by you in your role as mother, so help him out. Ask him to bring you a snack or a drink while you nurse. Say that the messy kitchen is driving you crazy—would he please wash the dishes? Suggest that he tell his mother that your milk is indeed good enough for your baby, that the doctor agrees, and that you really don't need any criticism right now, thank you very much.

It can be hard to ask for help during these weeks with your new baby. We women of the 21st century are convinced that we can do it all, or should be able to. We put up a strong front before our husbands because we want their respect and admiration, and then we end up struggling and resenting our spouses for not pitching in. We're victims of the image of capability we work so hard to create. Let down your guard a little, and share your feelings and your needs with your partner. He can't help unless he knows what to do. Let him know that you'd like him to take as much time off work as possible—that his simply being there means a lot to you.

Above all, tell your partner how much you appreciate his help. Tell him how important his presence was to you during the birth; most men don't realize the power of a loving touch or a steady hand holding the woman's during labor. Praise his growing fathering skills, and point out to him all the ways in which your baby responds to his father. Establishing a strong parenting partnership now will make all the difference in the years to come.

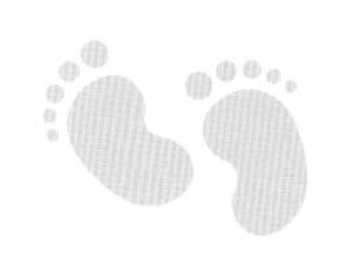

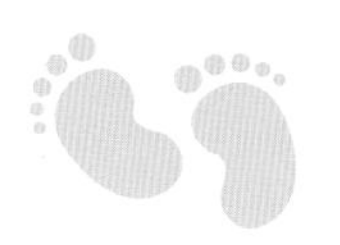

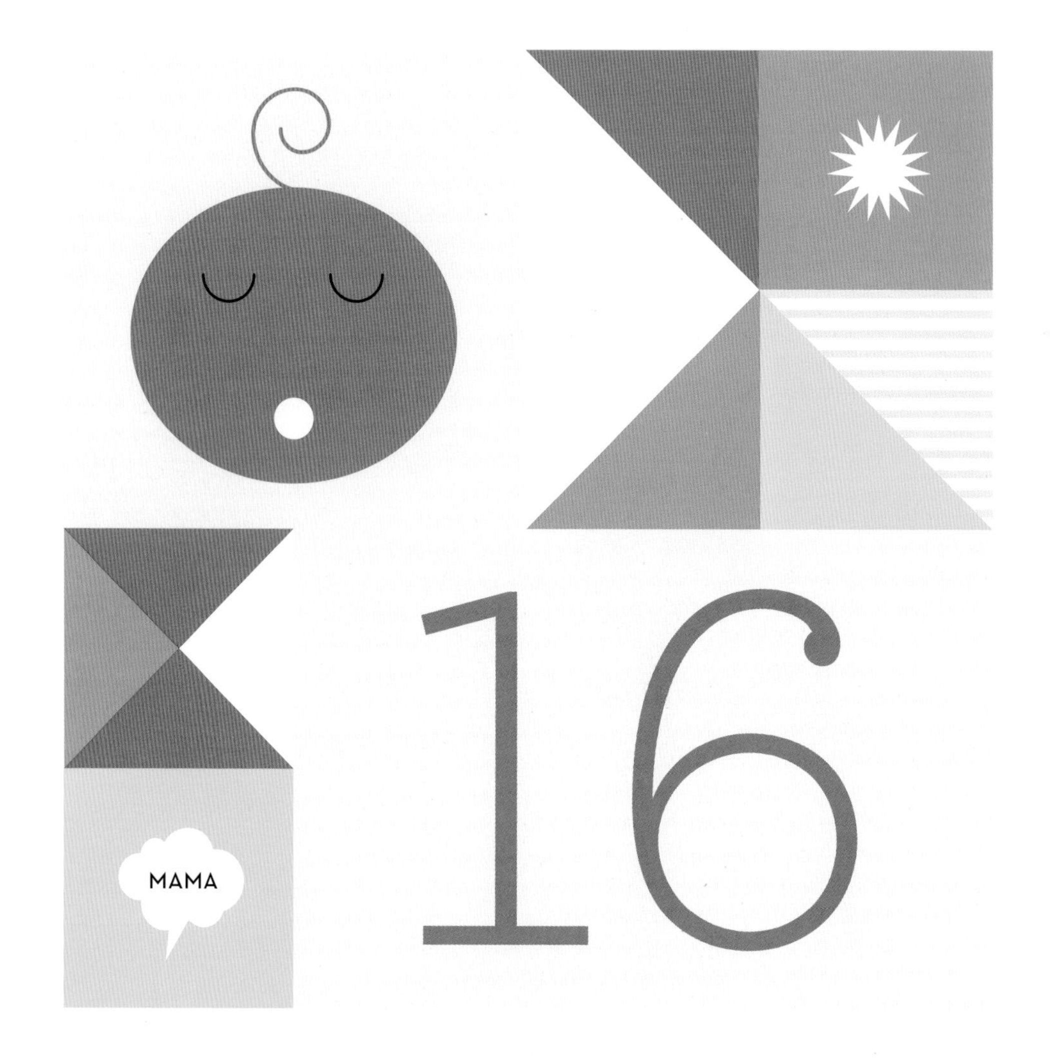
MAMA
16

It's All Right to Feel Like Crying

You have a beautiful new baby. Why are you crying?"

No woman who has ever had a baby would ask this question. Emotional ups and downs in the first weeks after birth are that common. Why wouldn't you cry sometimes? Your life is changing rapidly, you've been handed a huge new responsibility, and you can't even get an uninterrupted night's sleep.

It's important to understand the sources of "baby blues," those low feelings that attack vulnerable new mothers in the first days and weeks after giving birth. You'll have a better grip on what is happening to you if you understand the causes. You're not losing your mind; you're reacting to stressful circumstances.

First on the list are the physical realities of ending a pregnancy and becoming a mother. Your body undergoes tremendous change in a short period of time. The levels of pregnancy hormones drop suddenly; lactation hormones kick in. Once your body gets accustomed to the new hormonal levels, your moods and physical sensations will become more stable, but in the meantime these changes can contribute to crying jags.

Pain and discomfort from a cesarean incision or an episiotomy can lower your resistance to emotional stress, as can breastfeeding problems such as engorgement or intensely sore nipples. Lack of sleep, or even changes in your usual sleep pattern, can affect your ability to cope. These problems call for tender loving care, not just a slap on the back and an admonishment to "buck up and get on with it."

Some women experience a natural letdown after the elation of giving birth. You have spent months planning for this big event; after you come down from Cloud Nine, feelings of loss or anticlimax are to be expected. Yes, of course, you have your baby; but the day-to-day routine of baby care doesn't produce the same kind of emotional high that a wonderful childbirth experience will. So even though you now hold the object of all your preparation and labor, you may feel a little lost, and you may be chiding yourself for feeling this way. This is not what you expected.

That brings us to a major contributor to postpartum blues: the difference between our expectations of motherhood and the reality. Our culture paints a rosy glow around the ideal of a loving new mother, but does very little to help women live up to that picture. Page through one of those baby magazines lying around your house. Do the women in the pictures look tired or worn out? Even a picture of a mother looking worried, posed to illustrate an article about some typical dilemma, has the mother wearing clean clothes—without spit-up on her shoulder, or milk stains down her front. Her hair looks great—or at least clean, and what she's wearing not only fits her, it flatters her figure. Do you look like this right now?

We also expect mothers to be instantly sensitive to their babies' needs. What can be so hard about caring for little babies, if all they do is sleep and eat and sleep some more? And all husbands are devoted and intuitively understanding, right? The reality of life with a new baby never quite matches what we've been conditioned to expect. Even parents who have learned from the experiences of friends and family members get a jolt after their own babies are born. As with many things in life, it's easy to believe that only other people have problems.

If feelings of anxiety or depression hit you sometime in the first weeks after birth, the first thing to do is acknowledge and accept these emotions. Don't berate yourself for feeling this way. Most mothers, no matter how much they wanted their babies, no matter how good they are at caring for them, have moments of doubt and worry. Concern about now being a good-enough parent comes from love for your baby—you want her to have the best. Moments of self-doubt make you try harder to be the mother this baby needs. Tell yourself that you will be a good-enough parent, and remind yourself that this doesn't take a superhuman effort. You're the only mother your baby has, and she thinks you're wonderful.

It takes time to adjust to motherhood—time for you to learn to read your baby's cues, time for your body to settle into its new role as a food producer, time for your baby to grow up a little bit and show some appreciation for all your effort. You

The reality of life with a new baby never quite matches what we've been conditioned to expect.

also need time to discover yourself as a mother and make the necessary adjustments between your prenatal expectations and postpartum realities.

Meanwhile, take care of yourself. This means relying on others to do the non-baby tasks around your home for a while, or letting some things go. Your energy should be spent on your baby and on yourself. Take it easy; don't worry about the dust. Ask friends to bring you meals, or live on nutritious snacks and carry-out when you must. Eat well, but simply. A turkey sandwich and a pile of cut-up raw vegetables with an apple for dessert is just as nourishing as Thanksgiving dinner.

Pay attention to how you look. You don't have to look glamorous or put on makeup every day, but you do need to look nice to yourself. Get your hair cut; bring Dad or a friend along to hold the baby. Buy something new to wear that fits you right now and is easy to breastfeed in. Don't put off shopping for clothes, thinking that soon you'll be back to your usual size—you'll get depressed every time you open the closet door.

Get out of the house and get some exercise. No, this doesn't mean a high-pressure aerobics session or even a twice-a-week mother-and-baby exercise class (though you might enjoy this). Go for a brisk hour-long walk every day with the baby in a sling. Unless it's the dead of winter and extremely cold, your baby will be fine outdoors, snuggled close to you. This is a great way to get a fussy baby to sleep or to beat the afternoon blahs.

Being home alone all day with a new baby is mentally stressful. You need adult company. So take your baby and go places.

Moms, having repeatedly survived the postpartum period, I'd like to share with you a secret I've learned about new mothers.

Because they don't want to shake the supermom myth, they seldom ask for help, even when they need it. Husbands often assume that their wives don't need any help unless they ask for it. So ask, and be specific. Give your husband a list of things you need help with. Another problem is that when new mothers need a break they are often unwilling to release the baby to the father, unless he has proven himself capable of caring for the baby. But many fathers never get the chance to prove themselves. Here is a scenario I see quite often in my practice: A mother of a high-need baby gives so much energy to her infant that she has little or no reserve for herself. The father tries to help with the baby, but Mom hovers around, ready to rescue crying Baby from fumbling Daddy at the first millisecond of the cry. Instead of hovering over Dad and Baby, let your partner know that you are confident about leaving the baby in his care for a little while. Give them time and space to get to know each other, and they will get along just fine. And you will be less anxious, knowing your knight in shining armor will be there to hold the little bundle while you recharge.

—Bill

Ask friends over to keep you company. Attend La Leche League meetings, and look for other programs for mothers and babies in your community. Just talking with someone can lift your spirits for days.

Sometimes new-baby blues can grow into a full-blown postpartum depression, the kind that needs professional treatment. If you're experiencing incapacitating anxiety, lack of appetite, insomnia, mental confusion, inertia, or exaggerated fears, you should seek help quickly. Talk to your doctor for advice, or look for a support group for women experiencing postpartum depression (see Resources, page 202). Treatment for postpartum depression should not separate you from your baby or force you to stop breastfeeding. If you receive advice to the contrary, get another opinion.

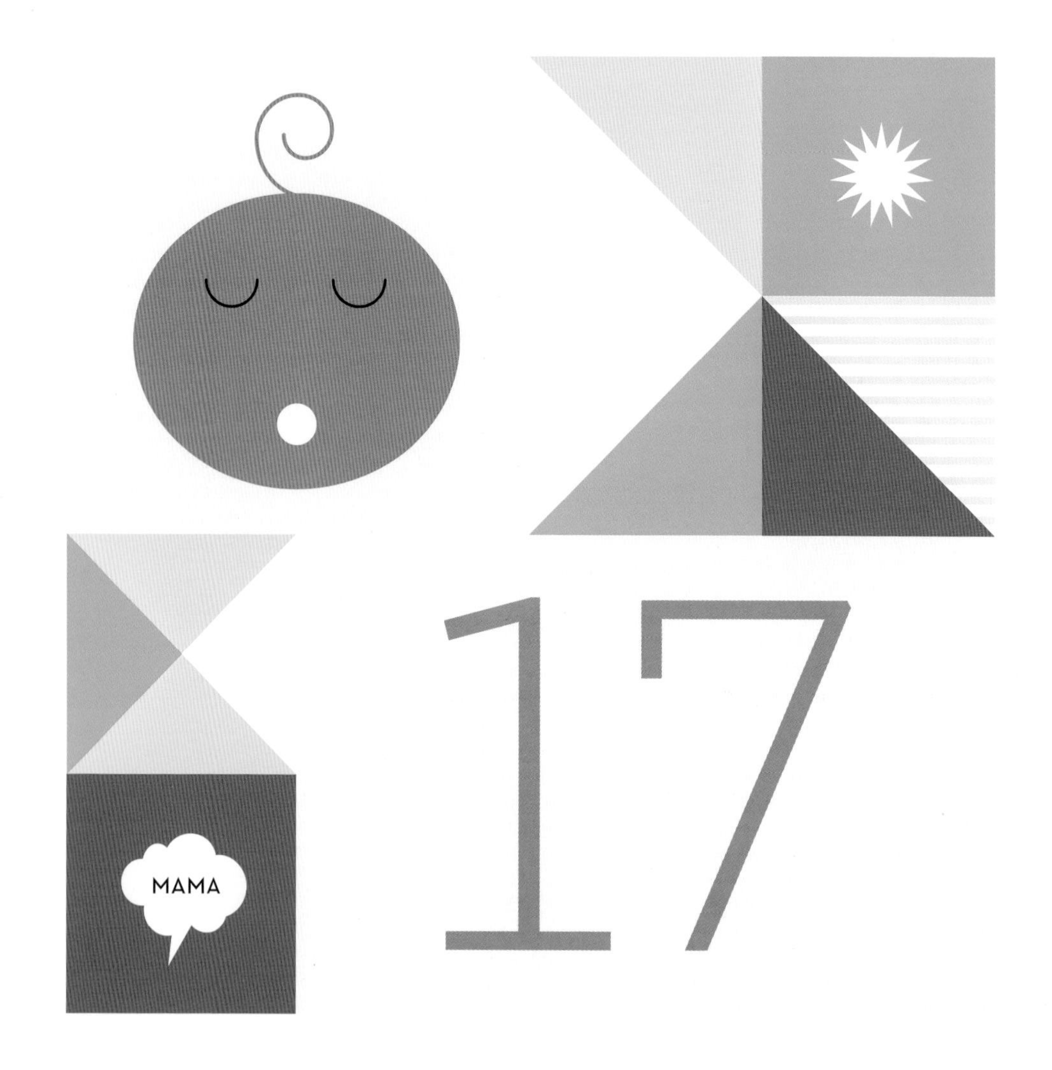
MAMA
17

Fathers Go On Being Husbands; Parents Are Still Lovers

Childbirth is not the end of the romance between you and your husband, but the new baby can make your relationship more complicated.

Your roles have multiplied; in addition to being husband and wife, you are now father and mother. You're no longer working to support just yourselves; you're breadwinners and caregivers. You're responsible! You are starting to think of yourselves as a family as well as a couple.

These changes happen in different ways and at different rates in men and women. At the moment, you may be far more focused on your mothering role than you are on being a wife. This is natural and understandable; the baby and your own hormones are propelling you in this direction. Your husband may be having a different experience. Even if he is very involved in baby care, he probably is not as concerned as you are with your infant's every sound or signal. His parenting anxieties may center on other matters: paying the mortgage, setting up a college fund, trying to be someone your child will feel proud of. This is a time of great change for him as well as for you, and he needs your support and reassurance just as you need his.

As you and your baby become finely attuned to each other, a great intimacy develops between you. It's made of communication, touch, warmth, love. You fill the baby's needs, and he gives good feelings back to you. Your partner may feel shut out of this inner circle. He doesn't have the physical bond of breastfeeding that you share with the baby, and he may be slower to develop the kind of sensitivity that makes baby care rewarding. He also may feel shut out of intimate relations with you. There's no time for all the things you used to do as a couple that reinforced your bond. You may both be dead tired, and possibly a little snappish. Sex seems too much to ask of a woman recovering from pregnancy and childbirth, especially when that woman has turned into someone's mother—whom he's not sure he even recognizes.

Men want sex and intimacy with their wives. They want romance (perhaps more than women do), and they want the appreciation and reassurance of their worth that comes from being part of a married couple. These male needs are not always apparent to a new mother, but they are important, and if you want your child to grow up having two parents, you'd better pay attention to them.

It takes a special effort to stay romantically involved with each other in the first months after your baby is born. Women often are not very interested in sex during this time (though some are). Part of the reason is hormonal. If you are breastfeeding, your body is telling you that you just had a baby and it's too soon to start another one. Psychologically, you're very absorbed in the relationship with your baby; it's hard to make room for someone else. Physically, you're tired and a little unsure of your postpregnancy body. Although the lack of sexual feelings during this time may surprise you, it is normal and temporary. If you do not respond to your husband's sexual advances as you once did, don't panic. You haven't fallen out of love. You haven't even forgotten how to be sexy. You're just going through a stage.

Your husband, however, is not in this same stage. He doesn't have all these reasons for not wanting sex. He needs you and the reassurance he gets from your sexual relationship.

What to do? Start by talking. Tell your husband how you are feeling, and explain that it is not his fault if you are not as interested in sex as you used to be. Reassure him that this is only temporary. Tell him what you need—holding, tenderness, sensitivity—in order to feel close. Tell him how much you appreciate everything he does for you and your baby.

Then, go ahead and give sex a try. You don't have to feel sexual to have sex, or even to enjoy it. It may be low on your list of priorities, but once you can relax (maybe with a back rub complete with massage oil?) and put other things—including your baby—out of your mind, you'll probably like it. It may take some time to learn how to shed the maternal feelings for a while and find the lover in you, but you can work this out, especially if

You haven't fallen out of love. You haven't even forgotten how to be sexy. You're just going through a stage.

you and your husband go slowly and show great care for each other's needs.

You may have to solve some practical problems. Once you have children, sex calls for a certain amount of sneaking around, especially if the baby is in your bed. If you can, nurse the baby to sleep in your arms and lay him down in the crib for the first part of the night. Or lie down with him and nurse him to sleep, tiptoe away, and find another part of the house that is suitable for lovemaking. Keep a towel handy if you tend to leak milk; oxytocin, the hormone that controls the milk ejection reflex, is released during sex as well as during breastfeeding. Use a water-soluble lubricant to counteract postpartum vaginal dryness. Experiment with different positions to find one that avoids putting pressure on areas still tender from stitches or tearing. If you feel too tired at night for sex, take a nap during the day when your baby is sleeping. Your husband would probably rather have a willing sex partner than a clean kitchen.

Sex benefits from romance, and romance also enlivens the rest of your relationship. Plan time to spend together. Plan "dates," even if these outings must include a breastfed baby. Dimly lit restaurants are perfect for nursing babies. Go early, or go late. Keep the baby awake during the soup and salad, then nurse her off to sleep before your entrée arrives. With the baby asleep in your arms (or in an infant seat at your feet, or next to you on the booth seat), you can linger over dessert and gaze into each other's eyes just as you used to. Go out to dinner now, while your baby is small; in a few months he will be grabbing everything in sight and dinner in a restaurant will not be relaxing.

You could also plan a special dinner for two at home. Dim the lights, get out the candles, and you'll never see the dust in the corners. Cook a simple meal together, or order carry-out and reheat it in the microwave on real plates when you're ready to eat. Put on some music. If you include the baby you won't have to worry about his waking up and spoiling the mood. You may have to take turns eating, but you'll be together, enjoying each other's company. Who knows where that could lead?

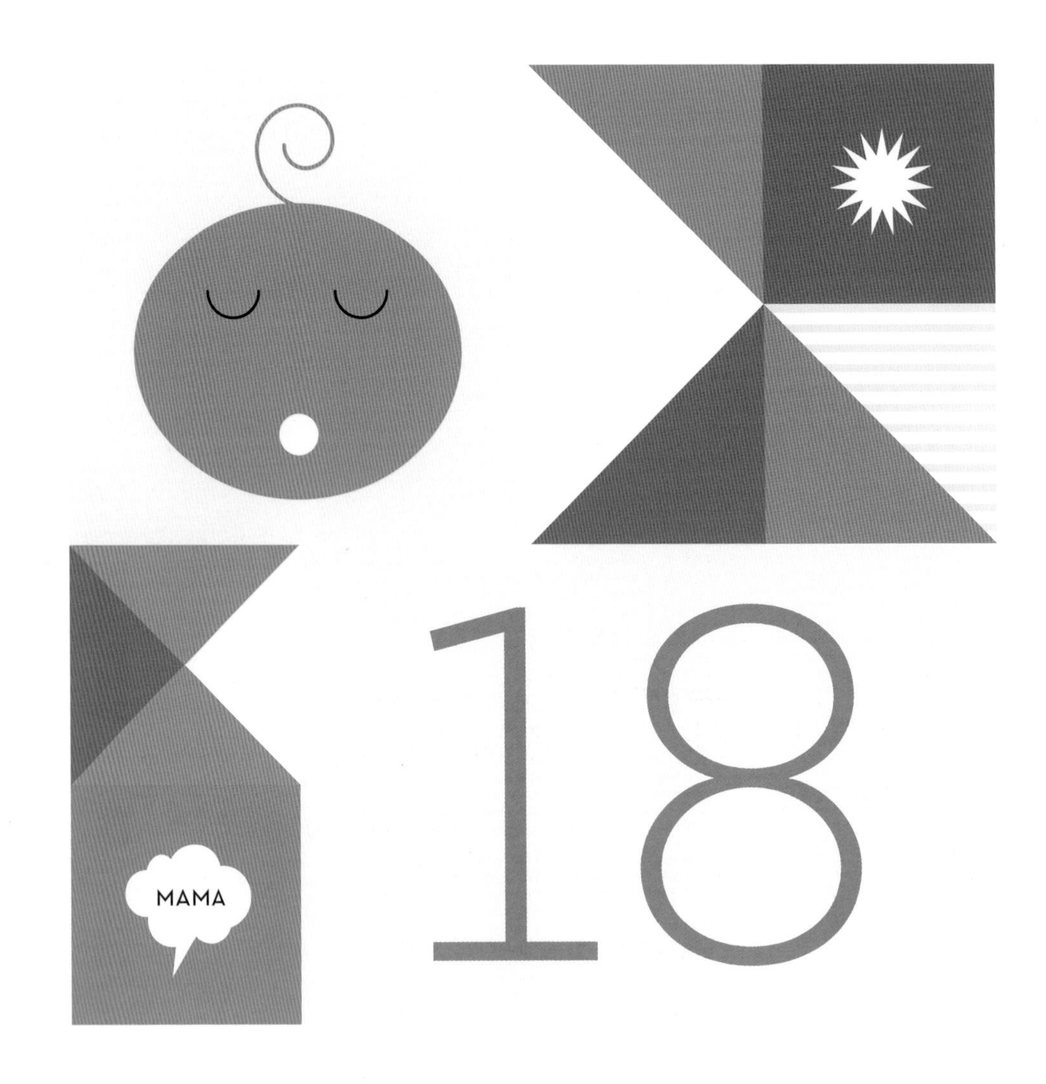
MAMA
18

Staying Home With Your Baby Can Be Practical and Rewarding

Nowadays, talking about mothers and work is like walking through a minefield. There are traps everywhere, and you'd better know the safe places to step if you want to avoid blowups. Families need the income, women need the stimulation, babies will be more independent—these are the things people say in support of the trend for mothers to return to their jobs after a few months' maternity leave. You won't read such remarks in the pages that follow.

Instead, I want to focus on the attachment that is growing between you and your baby. You are teaching her things, and she, in turn, is teaching you. She is learning to trust you, to tell you what she needs, and to be calm and happy inside herself. You are learning to understand her language, to trust her signals, and to find happiness in giving of yourself. These lessons are never exactly finished; they're part of an ongoing process that leads the two of you into a trusting and respectful relationship that will make parenting easier and more joyful in the years to come.

This attachment doesn't happen overnight, and it doesn't happen automatically. It takes time. You and your baby have to be together in order to learn from each other. And, unlike adults, who can schedule meaningful time together into a lunch date or a lazy Sunday afternoon, babies are completely spontaneous. You can't tell them to "hold that thought" for even a few minutes. You have to respond right then, or the opportunity is lost for both of you.

The main problem with employment outside the home is not the quality-versus-quantity-time issue, or even the difficulty of finding good child care. The problem is if you leave your baby for much of the day you are limiting your interactions with her. You will miss many of the moments in which you both could have made discoveries about each other. You won't love your baby any less if you return to outside employment while she is still quite young, but you will not know her in the same inside-out, "I-know-exactly-what-you're-thinking" kind of way. You also won't know as much about how to be her mother if you entrust many of the day-to-day details of that job to a substitute caregiver.

Being an unemployed mother does not guarantee that you and your baby will form a close attachment. You can be home all day and still make choices that interfere with this attachment—letting your baby cry it out, spending your time on various projects while your baby is cooped up in a crib or playpen. You can also be separated from your baby during work hours and make choices that maximize the attachment potential of the time you do spend together—continuing to breastfeed, babywearing, sharing sleep. But doing so will require a conscious effort on your part, and your sensitivity to your baby may lead you to discover that what she needs most is much more of you.

If you and your husband have decided that you must return to work for the good of the family economy, take another look. By the time you subtract the costs of working (taxes, child care, transportation, lunches, clothing, conveniences) from your

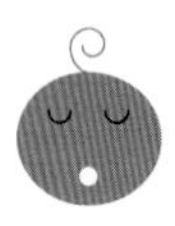

If you must go back to work, take the longest maternity leave you can.

paycheck, the amount on the bottom line may not be enough to justify the separation from your baby. (The long-term cost of separation is impossible to estimate.) You may be able to make ends meet in other ways. There are many options for mothers who need to earn money and still keep their babies close. The two-income daycare shuffle has become the standard for American families, but an amazing number of women are looking for alternatives and finding them. Consider working from home, starting a home business, getting a job that allows you to bring the baby along, doing home daycare for other employed mothers, or living more cheaply.

"But I'll go crazy at home!" Work fulfills many needs beyond that of a paycheck. You have friends at your job, order, purpose, challenges, a way to be part of what's going on in the world. It takes effort to create a new life for yourself at home, but here again you may have more options than you realize. Don't assume that you're "just not the type" to be a full-time, at-home mother. There is no one "at-home mother" type. Each of us shapes her mothering career in a way that suits her own personality and needs, as well as the needs of her children. If you have doubts about your mothering ability, if sometimes you think your baby might be better off in the hands of an experienced child-minder, it could be that you and your baby need more time together, not less. Think seriously about giving full-time mothering a try. You might contact the Family and Home Network, an organization started in 1984 for the purpose of supporting women who make this choice (see Resources, page 202).

If you must go back to work, take the longest maternity leave you can. You need this time to get tuned in to your baby. You and your baby should spend these weeks and months getting attached to each other rather than getting used to the idea of being separated.

Leaving a young baby with a substitute caregiver day after day is hard—and naturally so. When you're absolutely crazy about someone, you want to be with that person as much as possible. Mothers and babies are no exception. Don't be afraid to develop this kind of interdependent relationship with your baby. Whether you return to a job or stay at home full time, your baby's delight in your presence is a good thing. Encourage it.

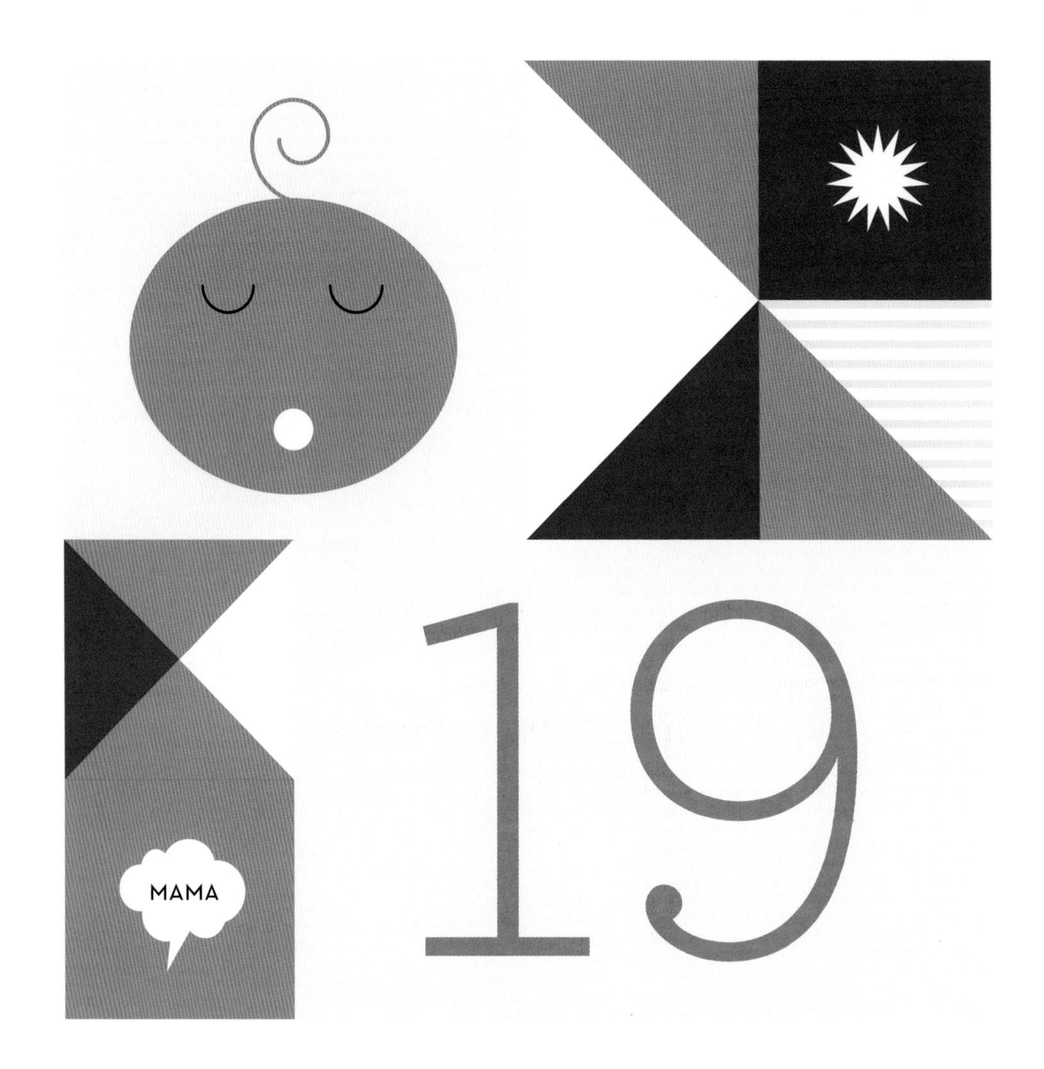
MAMA
19

If You Go Back to Work, You'll Still Be the Person Most Important to Your Baby

So you really must go back to work. How do you minimize the stress on your baby and yourself and maximize your time together?

The best thing to do is forget for now that you're going back to work. Take the longest maternity leave you can, and spend this time getting tuned in to your baby. The two of you should spend these weeks getting attached to each other rather than getting used to the idea of being separated. Let the love flow freely between you. Breastfeed following your baby's cues, keep him close to you day and night, and really enjoy each other.

Of course, forgetting about work is hard when you're worried about what will happen. It would be best to have certain things arranged well in advance, even before the baby's birth (such as finding a good babysitter), so that you *can* forget you're going back to work. You can decide in advance when you will introduce the bottle (more on that later) and then offer it once or twice a week so you won't have to worry that the baby will balk at the bottle for the sitter.

Look for a caregiver who understands your style of mothering and who will hold your baby a lot (maybe even wear him in a baby sling) and comfort your baby when he cries, just as you do. Although you want to stay at the top of your baby's list of preferred caregivers, he needs to be able to trust the one who cares for him when you're gone.

It might seem as if it would be better for the baby if you guarded against his wanting you above every one else, thus preparing him for the separation, but really it wouldn't be. Forging a strong bond now will help him through the times when you are gone. He will miss you, and he will be upset sometimes that you're not there, but having this kind of passion for his mother is important to his healthy emotional development.

On your end, don't let your feelings about leaving your baby prevent you from falling in love with him. Mothering demands a head-over-heels commitment. Don't think that you can carve out only a small space in your life and label it "baby." Until they're in the midst of motherhood, many women underestimate the intensity of the mother-baby bond. Confronting your passion for your baby can be frightening, because you must also think about just how hard it will be for you to leave him. One way of dealing with this emotional dilemma is to hold back and keep yourself from getting very attached. However, this approach hampers your ability to mother your baby and to know him really well. Don't be afraid of a healthy connection with your baby. The strength of your feelings will provide energy for the mothering challenges ahead and may even spill over into other areas of your life.

When it's time to start planning your return to work, look for ways to keep your connection with your baby strong. Continuing to breastfeed will maintain your biological attachment and nourish your emotional attachment. This may seem like a lot of bother—you'll need to pump your breasts at work, especially if your baby is less than six months old, in order to maintain your supply and provide breast milk for your baby when you're gone. Doing so is well worth the fuss. Pumping gives you a chance to think about your baby during your work day (looking at a picture of your baby is a good way to relax and get a lot of milk flowing) and to continue the satisfying feeling that you're giving your baby the very best nourishment.

For your baby, breastfeeding will be what makes Mom special. A substitute caregiver can bottle-feed, change diapers, soothe cries, and hopefully even love your baby, but only you can provide the wonderful closeness and contentment that comes with breastfeeding. Nursing is a wonderful way to celebrate your reunion at day's end. You'll both need and enjoy the time to sit down together and focus on each other before worrying about dinner or the night's chores.

You might want to start pumping and storing milk in your freezer a few weeks ahead of your return to the job (start earlier if you have too much milk in the early weeks). A reserve supply can take the pressure off you during times when your milk supply fluctuates because of your schedule or your baby's demands. Try pumping in the early morning, before your baby

When it's time to start planning your return to work, look for ways to keep your connection with your baby strong.

awakens, or midmorning, between feedings. Don't panic if you get only a small amount of milk at first. You'll get the knack soon, and you'll get more milk when pumping at work actually substitutes for feedings. I recommend renting a fully automatic electric pump for the best results and least stress. Contact La Leche League. (See Resources, page 205, for sources of information on purchasing and renting breast pumps.)

Should you get your baby accustomed to the bottle right from the start? Giving artificial nipples while your baby is still learning to breastfeed can lead to "nipple confusion" and other problems. It's best to wait about four weeks (longer if your baby has had a hard time learning to breastfeed) before introducing a bottle. When it's time to teach your baby to take a bottle, don't be anxious; make the process fun. Don't introduce the bottle when the baby is hungry, or you'll make him angry. Have the milk and the nipple warm, and keep the lessons short—start out with just a few sucks. Getting the baby to take a bottle may take some time. He may refuse to take it from you, since he knows the "real thing" is close by. If, after several sessions, the baby is still refusing the bottle, give this job to someone else—someone calm, patient, and experienced. After the baby accepts the bottle, a daily bottle feeding isn't necessary; one or two a week will be enough to keep him flexible.

When your maternity leave is nearly up, you may not feel ready to return to work and may want to try negotiating an extension. Some employers are understanding about this, others are less so. You're in the tricky position of having to balance commitment to your job and to your employer's needs with your commitment to your family. Try to see things from your employer's viewpoint as well as your own, but remember that you are the one who must speak up for your needs and your baby's.

Many sensible mothers start back to work on a Thursday instead of the traditional Monday. This gives them a weekend's

---

Not only is breastfeeding after you return to work good for your baby, it is beneficial for you.

Nursing your baby upon reunion is a wonderful way for you and your baby to reconnect. Many mothers also find that, upon coming home after a tiring day's work, sitting down and nursing their babies relaxes them. Breastfeeding lets those natural relaxing hormones work for you at the end of the day, when you need it. I can still remember how Martha and I juggled two professional careers (she as a nurse and I as an intern) while caring for our first baby. I remember shuttling Jim over to the hospital where Martha was working so she could breastfeed him during a break. If you truly believe breastfeeding makes a difference, you will find a way to continue.

—Bill

rest after only two days. Working part time for a while, if you can, will be easier on you and your baby. Take Wednesdays off for some midweek relaxation. Work six-hour days instead of eight. Bring work home and complete it with your baby nearby. Find a babysitter near your office rather than close to home so that you can visit your baby and breastfeed on your lunch hour, plus avoid being separated during the time you would otherwise spend driving.

When you are at home, put your baby first, above the cleaning and the errands and the adult agendas. Wear your baby, sleep with your baby, and expect some night nursing since you were apart all day (this helps keep up the milk supply). Expect your baby to stay up late at night just to be with you. Tell your caregiver that it's fine with you if the baby takes long daytime naps; this gives you more time to enjoy his company in the evening. Include your baby in everything you do outside of your job. Say no to other commitments. For now, you have your hands full with a job and a baby. The more time you spend with your baby when you're not working, the more connected you'll feel.

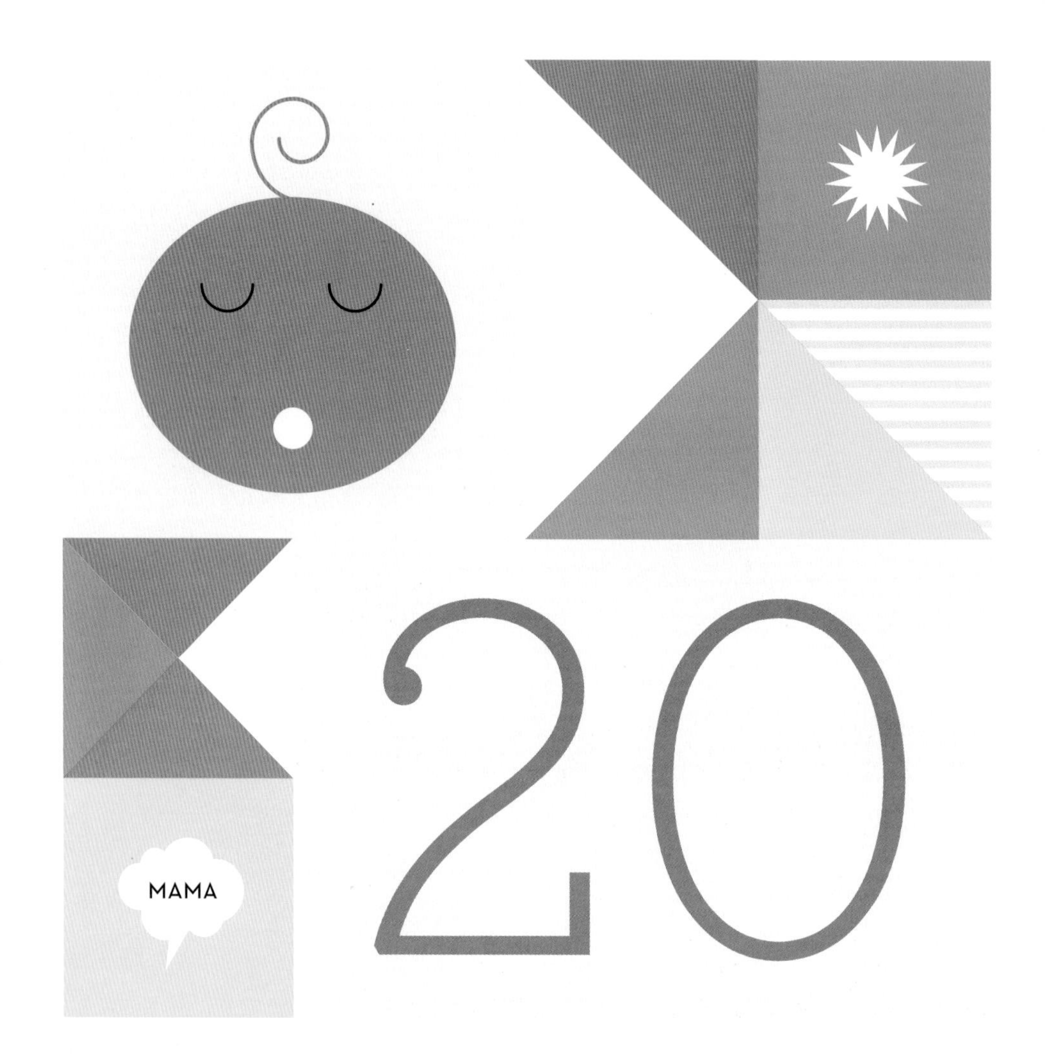
MAMA
20

Some Babies Are More Challenging Than Others

There are easy babies, and there are "high-need" babies, ones who ask a lot of their parents and complain until they get what they ask for. You'll soon discover if you have one of this type; they can wear a parent out very quickly.

High-need babies are supersensitive. They seem to need more help to cope with all the stimuli around them. They need to be in your arms all the time. They nurse frequently. They wake up when you set them down. They seem to need body contact even while they're sleeping. They never give you a break.

Having a high-need baby can change your feelings about motherhood. Whereas you may have imagined snuggling up peacefully with a contented, cuddly little one, you find yourself instead walking the floor as tired as you can be, trying to get a fussy, cranky baby to relax enough to doze off, if only for an hour or two. Your feelings about your baby may be less than loving at this point, and if you're like many mothers you tend to blame yourself: "What's wrong with me?"

Nothing's wrong with you. You're just stretched as far as you can go. Some women, because of their own inborn temperament and needs, reach this point sooner than others, but there's no shame in that. You do need to recognize, however, that you will have to make a few adjustments if you and your baby are going to thrive in the months to come.

The first shift you have to make is in what you are calling your baby. Difficult, demanding, fussy—these words all suggest you can't do much about the baby's behavior except resent it. The term "high-need" may serve you much better. It says, yes, your baby is a challenge—can you meet his expectations?

What exactly does "high-need" mean when it's applied to babies? Start with the assumption that a tiny baby's wants are the same as her needs, and remember also that crying is her only way of communicating. When the high-need baby fusses and complains, she is not doing it because she wants to bug her parents, or because she's spoiled, or because at her tender age she already has a quarrel with life. She *needs* something. This sounds obvious, but when you can't figure out what that something is or you're getting so tired that you just can't go

One of the main things our high-need babies have taught us is the concept of mutual giving.

The more we have given to our babies, the more they have given back to us. A mother of a high-need baby once confided to me, "This baby brings out the best and the worst in me." Although your special baby may extract every ounce of reserve energy from you, she is also helping you develop parenting skills that you may have never had the chance to acquire otherwise.

If you are blessed with a high-need baby, choose your advisors wisely. Surround yourself with positive people who affirm your parenting style. Avoid negative people and those who fear spoiling. Above all, don't take criticism personally. No one can understand a high-need baby unless he or she has had one.

—Bill

on, your frazzled nerves will leap to other conclusions. You'll decide that your baby is being unreasonable, rotten, and not at all the bundle of joy that you expected.

This is the moment at which you have to grab hold of the high-need concept, take a deep breath, and remember that you are the adult here and that you are dealing with another human being who is trying to tell you something. She is not just being petulant, and this is not a battle of wills that you have to win. Your job is to take care of this baby. This may mean your baby is at times inconsolable even if she is hardly ever out of your arms. But at least she knows, at a deep level, that you are there for her. Carefully reread Chapter 8 check with the doctor that your baby is healthy and is growing well, and, if you need more information on high-need babies, read our book, *The Fussy Baby Book* (see Resources, page 204).

Don't expect that you will be able to meet this baby's needs entirely on your own. This is the second adjustment you must make as the mother of a high-need baby. *You need help*. You need arms that can be there when yours are ready to give out. You need assistance with household chores and other tasks that compete with your baby for your energy. You need emotional support that affirms your efforts to give this baby what she needs—even if the baby doesn't seem very grateful. You may even need some help in understanding barriers within yourself that make it harder for you to recognize and cope with your baby's needs.

You can't give what you don't have. Your emotional tank can't run on empty. If you're struggling along, feeling miserable and alone while you try to mother a high-need baby, you're headed for trouble. If you don't take care of yourself, you can't take care of your baby. Ask for help. Talk to your partner, to family members, to friends. Have someone else hold the baby so that you can soak in the tub or get outdoors and take a walk. Reread Chapter 6 and double the emphasis on getting some help and taking care of *yourself*. Instead of thinking, "Why me?" ask yourself, "Who else?" Do some networking (through La Leche League, childbirth educators, midwives, your baby's doctor) to find other members with high-need babies, especially women whose babies are now a bit older. Remember that a few months from now, once your baby can do more physically, *things will be better*. I believe that every baby has a high need for attachment. It's just that some babies go about expressing this need with incredible intensity—they are not about to settle for a lower standard of parenting. This quality is actually a blessing in disguise; everyone in your family will operate at a higher level of sensitivity and responsiveness. So get out your Nikes and meet the challenge of your high-need "blessing," but don't try to go it alone.

MAMA
21

Continuing to Breastfeed Is Worth the Effort

Don't stop breastfeeding needlessly. Stay with it!

Most American mothers quit breastfeeding too early, by the time the baby is six months old, or much sooner. Very few are still nursing at a year. Ideally breastfeeding should continue until the baby is ready to stop, which is usually at some time well past her first birthday. As Antonia Novello, a former U.S. surgeon general, said, "It's the lucky baby, I feel, who continues to nurse until he's two."

"Yikes," you may say. "I'd never be able to breast-feed that long. I'm not even sure I'd want to."

There are often obstacles to overcome on the way to a successful, long-term breastfeeding relationship with your baby. Some of these have to do with feeling confident about breastfeeding, others with feeling good about it. As you become more comfortable with breastfeeding, you'll be less concerned about knowing when to stop. Before you wean your baby prematurely, consider the decision from several angles.

Ours is not yet a breastfeeding-friendly society. The clash between the needs of the breastfeeding mother and baby and the expectations of the world around them is often at the root of a mother's decision to wean. Giving up on breastfeeding may have nothing to do with a mother's ability to produce milk or with her baby's preferences. Other factors can work here, including a misunderstanding of how breastfeeding works and problems with fitting breastfeeding into a woman's lifestyle.

In many research studies, the most frequently given reason for stopping breastfeeding is not having enough milk. This can be puzzling to anyone knowledgeable about breastfeeding, since milk production works on a supply-and-demand basis. Normally, assuming your baby is latched on correctly and sucking strongly, your body will produce milk according to how much your infant nurses. The more milk he takes from the breasts, the more milk there will be. You don't have to wait for your breasts to fill up again between feedings. Although there are times when you will feel more full than other times, there is always milk in your breasts, and milk production is an ongoing process.

So why is it that many mothers feel they don't have enough milk when only a very small percentage of mother-baby pairs have anatomical problems that interfere with breastfeeding? First of all, as a new breastfeeding mother you have to learn to trust your body and your baby, and this isn't always easy. With bottle-feeding you see those ounces going in. You can add them up, and this basic arithmetic is reassuring to many mothers (and health professionals). With breastfeeding, you don't measure how much milk the baby is getting. You just trust the baby to nurse until his tummy's full, and to ask to nurse again when it's empty.

The crisis in confidence comes when a breastfed baby is asking to nurse very frequently. Surely, you think, he must be starving, but this probably isn't the case. He may be going through a growth spurt and is breastfeeding more often for a few days to fill his increased energy needs and to build up your supply. Or he may be nursing more often for other reasons—because he needs the comfort, because he's not feeling well, because he needs extra contact with you to get him over some developmental hump. He may just prefer a lot of small meals, or he may like having a “snack” a half-hour or so after he finishes “dinner.” Try thinking of his time at the breast as nurturing time instead of as feeding time.

Because it is so perfectly suited to a baby’s system, breast milk is digested faster than formula, and breastfed babies do get hungry more often. Don’t mistake frequent cues to nurse for a problem with breastfeeding. The problem is with all the baby-care advisors who have come to believe that the three- or four-hour feeding schedule that works for formula-fed babies should be applied to all babies. Oh, there may be some easygoing, undemanding breastfed newborns who nurse only six to eight times a day, but they’re not the norm. Breastfed babies usually nurse eight, ten, twelve times a day in the first few months, and those feedings are not evenly spaced around the clock.

There are ways to reassure yourself that your breastfed baby is getting enough to eat. First, have your baby’s weight checked around the fifth day after birth to be sure he is off to a good start. Although you can’t measure what goes in, you can keep track of what comes out. Look for at least six wet (not just damp) cloth diapers daily, four to five wet (that is, noticeably heavy) disposables. (It is harder to tell how much urine is in

Don't mistake frequent cues to nurse for a problem with breastfeeding.

a disposable diaper. I prefer using cloth in the early weeks for this reason, especially.) By age three or four days a breastfed baby will usually have three to five stools a day, although normal stools vary from two good-size ones daily to a little in the diaper (but more than a stain) at every feeding. Infrequent stooling in a breastfed baby less than two months old suggests that the baby may not be getting enough hindmilk, the extra-rich milk that comes at the end of the feeding. This baby needs to learn to nurse better. A lactation consultant or an experienced La Leche League leader can help you get this baby to improve his breastfeeding skills.

While frequent nursing is the key to having enough milk for your baby, frequent feedings may be perceived as one of the drawbacks of breastfeeding. You have to be there when the baby wants to eat. After a month or two of not being able to leave the house for more than two hours at a time, you may be thinking seriously about bottles. But there is another way to relieve cabin fever: Learn to nurse away from home. You can be a breastfeeding mother and still have a life.

You can breastfeed a baby almost anywhere. If you're careful, no one will even know what you're doing—although there's no reason to be embarrassed about it. There are a lot of ways to manage discreet breastfeeding in public. Wear clothes that are easy to nurse in. Use a baby sling and pull it up to cover the baby's head and your breast. Drape a blanket over your shoulder and over the baby. Practice ahead of time in front of a mirror or with a friend. When your baby wants to nurse when you're out somewhere, don't try to put her off. Her more insistent demands will only draw attention to your situation. Nurse her right away, and she'll stay happy and quiet.

It may take a while to feel comfortable nursing your baby in public places. But think about it: Women's breasts are displayed all over the place—in advertisements for automobiles, in fashion magazines, at the beach—and nobody blinks an eye. Why should anyone object to your using your breasts for their original purpose? Although some may insist that breastfeeding should be a private matter, babies' need to nurse frequently argues against this. Breastfeeding mothers should not have to be second-class citizens, forever hiding out in bathrooms to meet the needs of their babies.

Even a return to work does not have to mean the end of breastfeeding. You will have to pump your breasts when you are away from your baby in order to maintain a good milk supply and provide breast milk for your baby while you are away. But you can continue to breastfeed and enjoy warm and snuggly reunions with your baby at the end of your workday.

If your family and friends are uncomfortable with your breastfeeding, it really helps to get support. Attending La Leche League meetings is one of the best things you can do to help yourself breastfeed longer. Being with other breastfeeding mothers can help you see breastfeeding as normal, not the thing that may be making you an oddball in your family or neighborhood. Spending time with other breastfeeding families will help you realize the full rewards of breastfeeding: not just the better health and nutrition it affords your baby, but the joy and closeness it brings to your relationship. With positive attitudes toward breastfeeding, you'll be able to overcome any problem that comes your way.

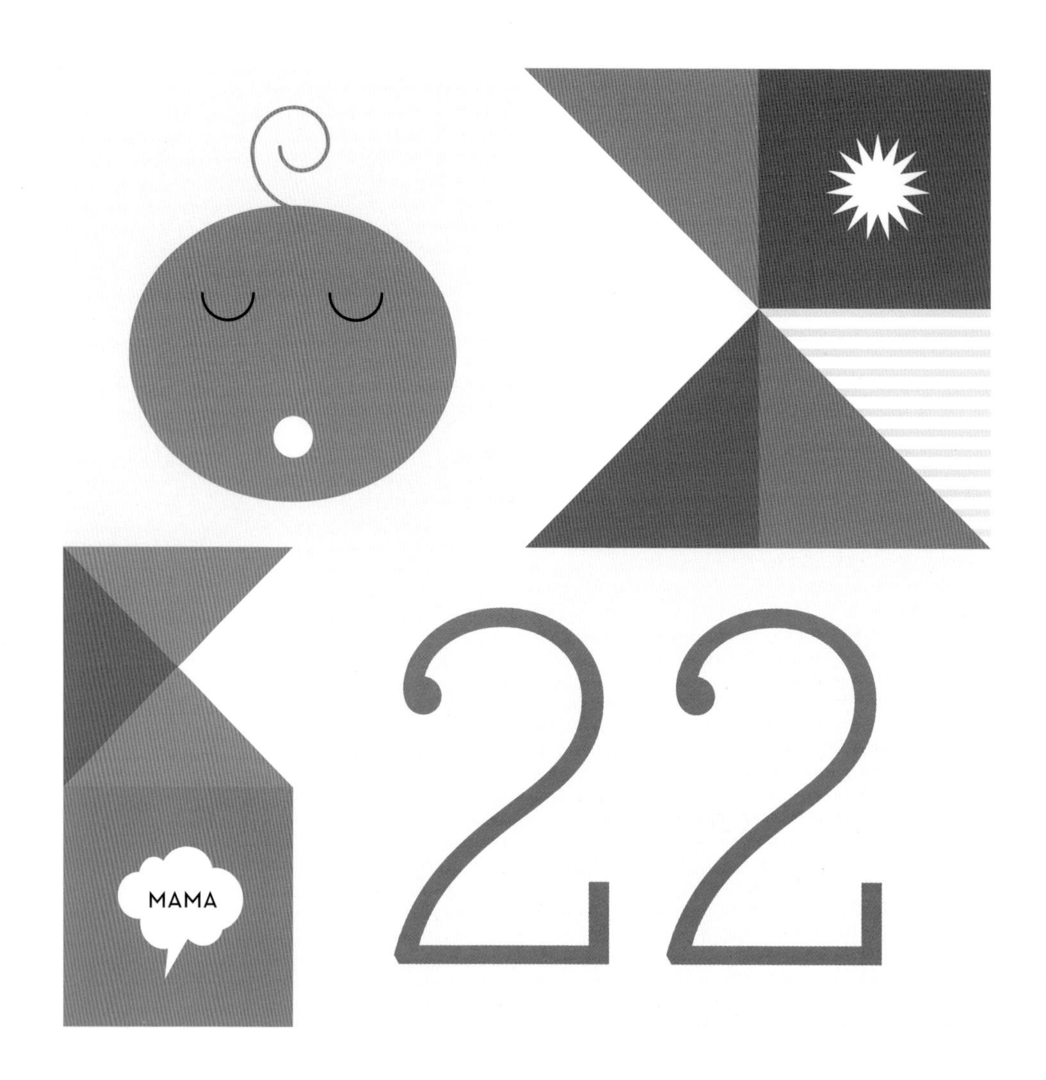
MAMA
22

You Are the Expert on Your Baby

When you have a baby, you discover very quickly that everyone—friend or stranger—wants to give you advice, whether you ask for it or not. It's always open season on new parents.

Some of this advice is actually helpful. Experienced parents can provide you with all kinds of useful information—be it where to shop for shoes, how to get the laundry done, or what to do when your baby cries. If you meet some trustworthy advisors as you journey into parenthood, treasure them and turn to them when you need their particular brand of expertise.

However, not all advice is created equal, and not all of it will be right for you. It's not terribly hard to figure out which advice to disregard. Advice that feels wrong to you—that makes you say to yourself, "Oh, I couldn't do that with my baby"—or that is aimed to put distance between you and the baby is better left unheeded. The intuitive part of you, the part that knows and feels for your baby, will be very uneasy if you use this kind of "help."

Baby-rearing advice can have an unfortunate side effect. It can undermine your confidence as a mother. Your heart may be telling you one thing, but your mother, mother-in-law, sister, and best friend all disagree. The voice of your heart can fade away when it has to compete with the noise from the crowd. It's hard to feel right about the way you do something when some very experienced people think you should do it differently.

This is through no fault of your own. Because you love your baby so much, you want what is best for her. For the sake of

The awesome responsibility of taking care of a tiny, helpless human being humbles a parent.

her long-term happiness, you're willing to try almost anything, whether it's recommended by a book, a doctor, or the old lady you met at the post office. The awesome responsibility of taking care of a tiny, helpless human being humbles a parent. As much as you try and as strong as your own convictions are, the importance of what you are doing strikes fear in your heart.

Even if you're new at the parenting business, you can trust your convictions about what is right for your baby, as long as you are reading her cues and learning to be responsive to her needs. You may have to throw off some preconceptions of your own along the way ("All babies do is eat and sleep."), but the time you spend with your baby makes you the expert on this unique individual, sometimes in ways that defy logic.

This doesn't mean that if you are an intuitive, responsive mother you won't feel shaken by advisors who tell you that you're doing it all wrong. You will wonder at times if you are doing the right thing, especially when it flies in the face of the latest article in the parenting magazine. If the advice comes from people who are important to you, such as your mother or a good friend, you may feel lonely sticking to your own convictions. When you're new at something, you want the approval of people you care about and respect. It can be hard to go your own way without support.

Dealing with unwanted advice and criticism is a major problem for new parents. Many emotional issues are involved, not the least of them your need to establish yourself as an independent adult, capable of handling the responsibilities of parenthood. The temptation to argue is powerful; yet you hesitate lest you hurt the relationship, since this is such an emotional time for you. You may not even know what you'd say. Confrontation is not a good way to handle an already touchy situation.

Keep in mind that your advisors feel they have your best interests at heart. They care about you and your baby and feel they should do something to make things easier for you. Acknowledge this and thank them—"I know you think this must be hard for me. Thanks for caring, but I would be a wreck if I let the baby cry." Give them some other way to help you: "Maybe you could bring dinner over one night this week?"

Along with good intentions, baby-care advice is often mixed with a need for advisors to have their own parenting experience affirmed. If your mother did not choose to breastfeed, she may be very threatened by your decision to breastfeed your baby. She may feel as if you're showing her up, making her feel that she wasn't a very good mother to you. A couple whose irritable baby was left to cry it out at the advice of some so-called expert may secretly envy your calm, quiet in-arms infant and regret that they did not take this route themselves, even as they lend you the book that they followed. This is no time for you to crow about your new, improved, psychologically better way of nurturing an infant. Realize instead that these people were trying to do the best for their babies in their situations and with the information available to them. If you can, find something you genuinely admire about their parenting, and talk about that instead. You'll soon learn whom you can share ideas with—stick to the people you can count on to be supportive.

Sharing information is a good way to defuse criticism. A few facts work wonders: "Because it's the perfect food, breast milk digests quickly and babies get hungry sooner," or "Babies who are held a lot in the first six weeks tend to cry less later on." It's

One of our goals in this book is to help you create a style of parenting that brings out the best in your baby and yourself, and makes you your own expert on your baby.

In my decades in pediatric practice, I have noticed that mothers and fathers who practice attachment parenting are more likely to know their babies better; they are more observant of their babies, and they respond more sensitively and appropriately to their babies' cues. The ability to read and know your baby can bring you great comfort and confidence, as well as simply help you to enjoy your baby more.

—Bill

hard to argue with statements of fact. You can also rely on the statement "Every baby is different" for getting advisors off your back. Or try, "We know our baby, and this works for us." Then go on to a new topic, like the weather.

What to do about crying and where the baby should sleep are the two lightning rods for criticism of baby-tending styles. As usual, most people's concern is for the baby to become independent. If you hold your baby a lot to comfort his crying, expect that some people will say you're spoiling him and he will never want to be anywhere else. Just remember that babies don't develop along logical lines. Filling their need for closeness to parents actually prepares them for independence, not for a lifetime of sticking to mother. Sleeping with your baby draws similar comments. People have a difficult time grasping the idea that early dependence fosters later independence. Maybe their own sense of independence is not well grounded in trust and security.

Dealing with criticism as a new parent requires that you act in a mature manner. You have to be willing to tolerate other viewpoints and not have to prove yourself right. This isn't always easy when you're feeling vulnerable, unsure of yourself, or just plain tired. But, remember, you truly are the expert on your baby. Just a few days of being with her constantly has earned

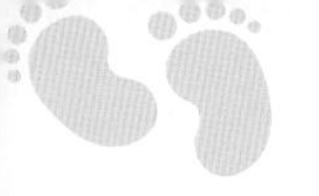

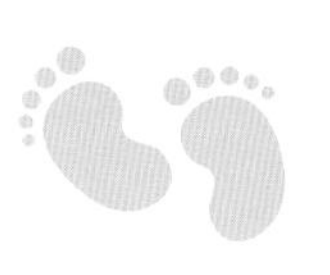

you the right to call yourself that. So follow your heart and your baby's cues. In a few months, your content and happy baby will be the best argument in favor of all you are doing as a responsive, intuitive parent. Your critics will have to admit you're doing something right, and you will feel that your confidence in yourself as a mother is justified.

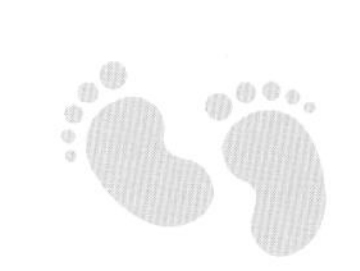

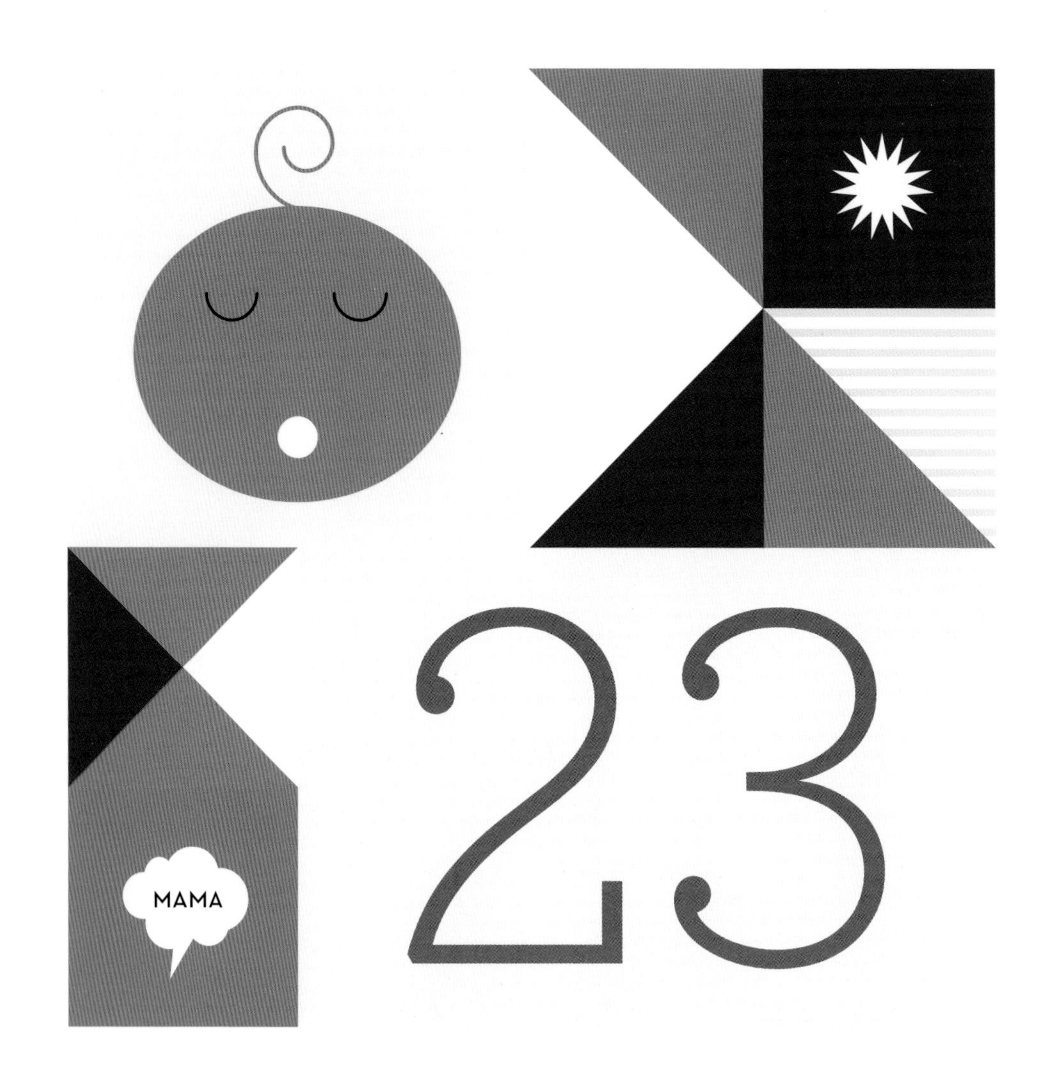
MAMA
23

You Need People to Lean On

To defend yourself against attacks of self-doubt, loneliness, and worry, get some support. Don't shut yourself away from the rest of the world.

Mothers who are home with small children have a higher than average incidence of depression. One of the causes of this is isolation. Long hours with no other adults to talk with and the persistent demands of an infant to attend to can take a toll on your emotional well-being. This is not how things are supposed to be.

Imagine a century and a half ago, when most people lived in small communities and helped each other out. Members of the extended family lived nearby, if not in the same house, and shared large tasks, cared for the sick, and helped with the children. Husbands and fathers worked in the barn or in the fields or in a shop downstairs, and came back to the home for meals at midday. There were usually other women close by—friends, sisters, mothers, and aunts—to talk with and to learn from.

Contrast this scene with that of the modern mother. She and her husband have their own place. There may be family members nearby, in the next suburb, perhaps, but probably not next door. The nearest relatives may live a thousand miles away. If this is her first baby, the mother's friends may all be working women, with a different lifestyle and different interests. She may not even know her neighbors, and few, if any, of them are home during the day. She shops in large chain stores, where no one recognizes her from one visit to the next. After her husband kisses her goodbye in the morning, she may not talk to another adult until he comes home at night.

To survive the stresses of early parenthood, you need to shape your life to be more like the first example. You must build yourself a support system. It can include all kinds of people who fill different needs for you. Having friends to lean on will make your life as a mother easier and more enjoyable, more rewarding.

Husbands are usually the most important source of support for mothers, but they should not be the sole suppliers. Sometimes it really helps to be able to talk with another woman, especially another breastfeeding mother, or someone with many years of experience as a parent. Sometimes the best source of support is someone who has a baby the same age as yours and who is facing similar challenges.

There are a lot of ways to build a support system; some potential sources of support are just waiting for you to tap. One place to start is with the other women from your childbirth class. Dig out their phone numbers and arrange a reunion. You'll have birth stories to share, along with baby-care struggles.

La Leche League is the grandmother of support groups for new mothers. League meetings are more than a source of information on breastfeeding; they also provide support for responsive mothering. You'll be surrounded by women who are convinced that attending sensitively to their babies' needs is the best way to mother. You'll also get to watch more experienced mothers and learn from their example. (To find a La Leche League group near you, dial 877-452-5324, or visit the Web site at www.lalecheleague.org.) If you feel uncomfortable at the meeting you attend (the leader is too radical, the other mothers are overbearing, or you just feel you don't fit) try another meeting or even another group nearby before you give up on this source of support. Each group (even each meeting) has its own flavor depending on the personalities involved. You'll want a group you can relate with. The good feelings you get from a La Leche League meeting can keep you going for weeks.

Your community probably has other resources for mothers and babies. Mothers' support groups may meet at a local church, at the "Y," or at a community center. Look into these, and give them a try. If one group doesn't suit you, perhaps another will. Signing up for a mother-baby exercise program is another way to meet other women with new babies. You may be able to find other parents among former work associates, people you already have something in common with. And, who knows, maybe on one of your many walks you'll meet a woman who lives just a few blocks away, and she might even be using a baby sling, too.

When you find someone with whom you feel at ease, who shares your parenting values and some of your other interests, put some effort into striking up and continuing the friendship. Make plans to take a walk together one morning or to share a simple mother-baby lunch. You may find that for some kinds of support you turn to one group of people, and that at other times different friends fill your needs.

Don't sell short the place of your mother, mother-in-law, or other family members in your support system. Even if you don't agree with them on every baby-care issue, they do love you and your baby. If all of you can agree to disagree at times, you may actually learn things from one another. Many women find that their relationships with their own mothers grow and deepen when they have children of their own.

Your support system can even include books, magazines, and Web sites that help you feel good about your style of parenting. See the online La Leche League catalog for books that support responsive mothering. Three excellent parenting magazines are *Mothering*, La Leche League's *New Beginnings*, and *BabyTalk* (see Resources, page 203). Remember, you don't have to believe or accept everything you read. Be especially cautious about what you read on the Internet. Avoid books, magazines, Web sites, chat rooms, or e-mail lists that cause you to doubt your own intuition about your baby.

Adjusting to being a mother is hard. It is a major life transition. A support system can make all the difference in how well you come through the changes.

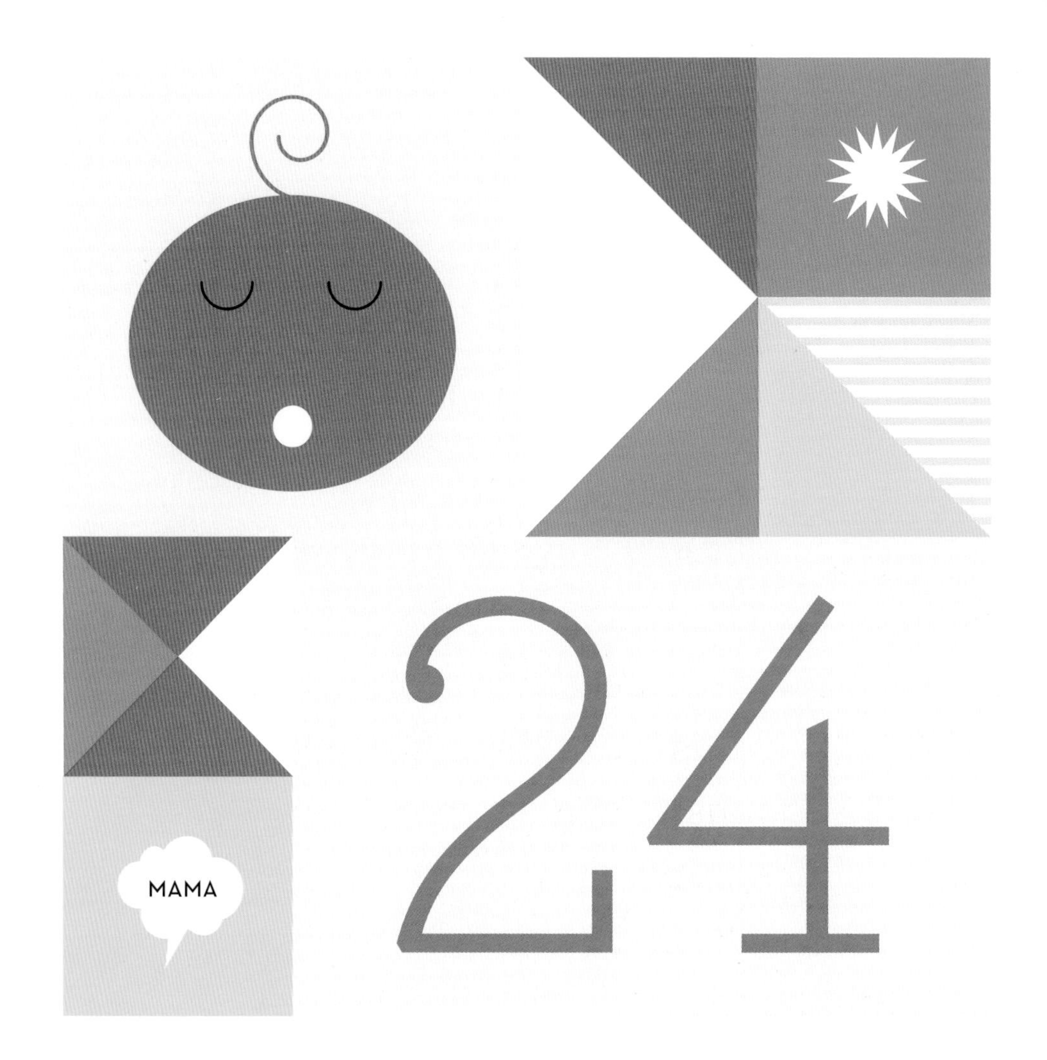
MAMA
24

You Don't Have to Be Perfect

Some women are born perfectionists, or they acquire this quality early in childhood. Everything must be just so, and they work very hard to get straight A's, to land an important job, to marry an impressive man, to create a beautiful home.

Other women become perfectionists when they have children. Love, along with other motives, drives them to it. They want their children to have the best, to have the things they never had themselves, to have the mother they wish they had. They struggle to do everything "right," believing that this will ensure their children's health and happiness in the years to come.

They want their babies to have the best start in life, so they eat well during pregnancy. They plan for a perfect labor and birth that follows a predetermined timetable. They breastfeed because they know it's the best. They devour parenting books, and panic if their baby isn't measuring up to the developmental progress of her same-age cousin.

There's a high price to pay for perfection. You can drive yourself crazy trying to be a perfect mother, even of a tiny newborn, let alone several rambunctious school-age kids. And even if you do everything absolutely by the book (even this book), there is no guarantee that your kids will turn out the way you want. In fact, perfection is harmful to children, for perfect children never have the opportunity to learn how to accept their mistakes.

The good news is you don't have to be perfect. You don't have to be right all the time. You don't have to agonize constantly over what's best. All you have to be as a mother is good enough, good much of the time, good overall. What counts is the prevailing feeling in your relationship with your baby, not the play-by-play tally of runs and errors.

Take breastfeeding, for example. Human milk is best for babies, and it's a fortunate baby whose mother chooses to breastfeed her. However, breastfeeding should not be a grit-your-teeth-and-get-through-it experience, undertaken only because of a list of scientific advantages. Even if you start out breastfeeding motivated only by recommendations from experts, you soon discover that a desire to be perfect is not a strong enough motivation when problems arise. Fortunately, nature has built in some safeguards. Breastfeeding is relaxing and enjoyable for most women, and when you discover this for yourself, you can let go of the "I'll bear it for my baby" attitude. Everything about feedings, including your baby's reactions, will become much more natural, good enough to help your baby thrive and grow and keep you content and confident. (If this doesn't happen, and you truly are miserable breastfeeding, I believe it is better for you to bottle-feed so your baby can see a happy face most of the time. You may find breastfeeding easier next time, if you have another baby.)

It's a good idea to eat well while you're breastfeeding, mostly for the sake of your own health and well-being. But say you're not perfect—you go on a junk-food binge one afternoon and

Although a good mother tries to help her baby when she's crying, even a "perfect" mother can't prevent crying altogether, and it would hurt her baby's emotional development if she attempted to.

polish off the potato chips and the Oreo cookies. Have you blown it? No, of course not. Your milk is still wonderfully nutritious for your baby, even if you didn't follow a perfect diet. Tomorrow is another day, and a salad will probably appeal to you at lunchtime.

Crying is another area where you should let go of ideas of perfection. You won't always be able to help your baby stop crying. Responsive mothering doesn't mean that you squelch a baby's negative emotions. You soothe and support, and most of the time this stops the crying. When it doesn't, you continue to comfort your baby and try new ways of helping her, but you don't blame yourself for her hurts and sensitivities. Although a good mother tries to help her baby when she's crying, even a "perfect" mother can't prevent crying altogether, and it would hurt her baby's emotional development if she attempted to.

You don't have to have a perfect house, either, whether you or your husband thinks you should. Being comfortable with some untidiness may take some practice; but when you're devoting most of your time to caring for your baby, lowering your housekeeping standards is not only inevitable, it's healthy. If you're spending all your available non-mothering time scurrying around after dust bunnies, washing windows, or finally repapering the bathroom, you'll quickly run out of energy.

You'll become a crabby person who is obsessed with streaks on the mirror and couch cushions still out of place from the last nursing session. Soon there will be a conflict over how you spend your time: cleaning and polishing versus caring for and playing with your baby while recharging your own batteries. Now, really, which do you think is more important?

It's not that you should never clean; some order is necessary for your sanity. Just keep the ideal of the perfect house in its place. You may need to encourage your husband to lower his standards, take on a bigger share of the work, or both. You should both remember that all the gorgeous homes you see in magazines and all the perfectly kept yards you drive past on the way to the grocery store probably don't belong to people who are trying to juggle housekeeping and caring for a new baby. Try to take the long perspective. Someday your children will grow up and move out and you can have a perfect house—if you still want one. No one on her death-bed ever wished she had spent more time cleaning her house, and no one on her death-bed ever regretted spending too much time with her children.

If your perfectionist tendencies are surfacing now that you've become a mother, relax and ease up on yourself. Chances are, you're doing the best that you can do, given the circumstances of the moment and the resources available to you. Don't fall into the trap of thinking that you're not good enough. If you are enjoying your baby and feeling that you really know and understand her, you've definitely got the hang of motherhood. Savor each moment of your baby's life for what it is, instead of thinking of something more that could be done. If you stay tuned in to your baby most of the time, you'll be the mother that your baby needs—a far better thing to aspire to than some distorted vision of perfection.

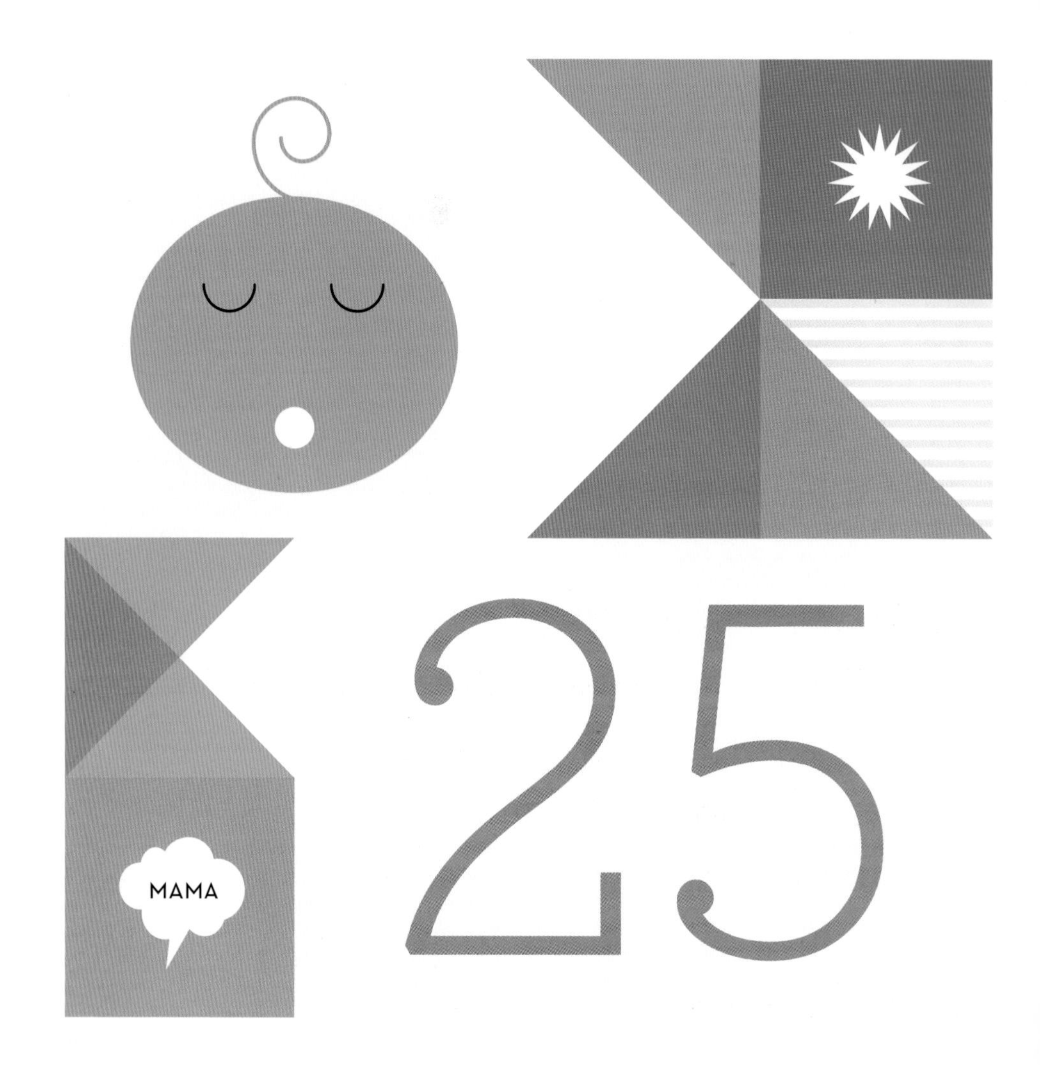
MAMA
25

How You Mother Your Baby Does Make a Difference

Mothering in the 21st century has become a tricky business. We can take our babies' survival pretty much for granted, and in this way we differ from all the mothers who have come before us. Instead we worry about whether our babies will grow up to be happy and productive, a more complicated issue.

Nobody yet has scientifically tested and perfected a parenting system that guarantees children will turn out okay. Much of the research focuses on what goes wrong, rather than what goes right, and psychologists from Freud onward have often laid the blame on mothers. This creates a lot of anxiety, as mothers struggle to raise psychologically healthy children. Mothers often feel that the stakes are high on everything they do, and the possibility of making serious mistakes makes the job of parenting seem frightening.

In reaction to Freud, there's another school of thought that suggests that mothers aren't all that critical to their children's psyches. Children need dependable caregivers, yes, but these are more or less interchangeable, and group care not only is satisfactory, it also makes children independent at an earlier age. Babies do prefer their parents, but they really don't need all that one-on-one attention that goes along with traditional mothering. It's interesting that these theories have evolved at a time when more and more mothers of young children are in the workforce.

So where do you fit in? How important are you, a responsive, nurturing, trustworthy mother, to your baby's development? How do you know if you're making a difference?

In the parenting business, science often fails us. It's hard to study behavior that is as complicated as mother-and-infant interactions, much less relate these interactions to how children behave and feel years later. “Experts” speculate, spinning advice out of tiny threads of evidence, but who really knows?

For babies, attachment parenting includes closeness right from birth, responding sensitively to cries, baby-wearing, sharing sleep, and breastfeeding.

I believe that experienced parents—parents of children who are turning out well—have the answers. Bill and I have talked to thousands of wise and seasoned mothers over the years, and while we don't pretend that this is a scientific sample, we do feel confident about relaying what we've learned from all these families. We believe that how you mother your children makes a difference in the kind of people they become.

The mothering advice that we have given in this book reflects a style that we call attachment parenting. For babies, attachment parenting includes closeness right from birth, responding sensitively to cries, babywearing, sharing sleep, and breastfeeding. The involvement of the father, both directly with the baby and in support of the mother, is also important. These practices together make up a very nurturing style of baby care, one that yields a wonderful sensitivity between mother and child. The mother understands what the baby is thinking, most of the time, and the baby responds well to the mother's care. Babies who experience attachment parenting rarely need to cry to get their needs met (though they may cry plenty when something hurts or bothers them), because they can communicate in other, more subtle ways. Mothers who nurture in this style feel confident that they are doing the right things for their children, because they feel they can perceive their babies' needs, and because their babies are happiest when they are most responsive. Even high-need babies can be mellowed by this style of parenting into children who are fun to be with.

There are long-range benefits to attachment parenting. As a baby cared for this way turns into a toddler, he is easy to manage. His mother has a pretty good idea of what he is trying to do or say, so the young explorer is less likely to get terribly frustrated. Since he trusts his mother and wants very much to stay in her good graces, a word of warning or some creative redirection from her is often all that's needed to head off problem behavior.

When you bring home a new baby, remember you are modeling parenting for your older children. Consider that you are bringing up someone else's future husband or wife, father or mother.

The parenting styles children learn are the ones they are most likely to follow when they become parents. Here is an example of how modeling affects children: A mother brought her newborn, Erin, and her two-and-a-half-year-old, Tiffany, into my office for checkups. During her examination, Erin began to cry. Tiffany rushed to her mother, pulled at her mother's skirt, and exclaimed, "Mommy, Erin cry; pick up, rock-rock, nurse!" This little child had just described responsive parenting according to her mother's model. When Tiffany becomes a mother and her baby cries, what do you imagine she will do? She won't consult a book or call her doctor. She will intuitively pick up, rock-rock, and nurse.

—Bill

As children of attached parents grow older, the benefits continue. These kids internalize their parents' sensitivity toward them. They have an inner sense of what is right and are bothered when situations violate their values. They know themselves well and can remain true to their own character in the midst of a crowd going in another direction. They are compassionate and understanding with other people. Having learned intimacy from their early closeness with their parents, they go on to establish and maintain healthy relationships with other people. They bring their parents joy and pride.

So, are you important to your baby? Yes, you are. You as his mother know him best and are the person he trusts most and will look to for guidance in the months and years to come. You are his window to the world and his faithful interpreter of what is going on inside him. Your relationship is built on a long history of knowing each other, a history that begins even before birth. Because this relationship is grounded in love and trust and many small interactions, it can tolerate mistakes and misunderstandings. No single moment is critically important. What counts is the harmony that is developing between you.

So relax and enjoy your baby. Although this special time in your life is full of worries and adjustments, it is also full of wonder. You have much to look forward to. Being a mother can enrich every corner of your life. Get ready for a marvelous journey.

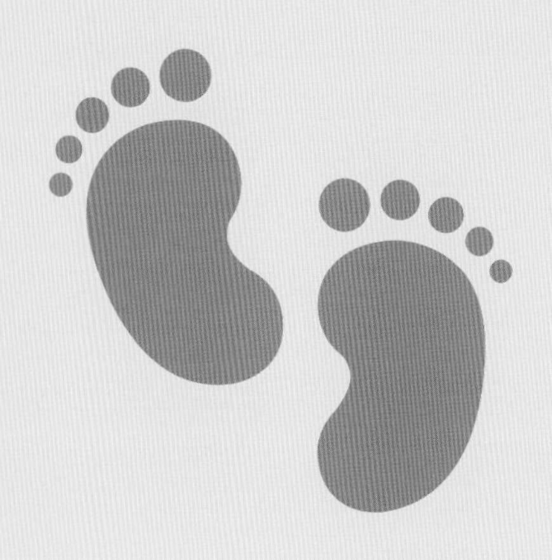

Resources

Organizations

Attachment Parenting International (API)

API promotes parenting practices that create strong, healthy emotional bonds between children and their parents.

www.attachmentparenting.org

Doulas of North America (DONA)

The leader in doula training, certification, and continuing education.

www.dona.org

Family & Home Network

A non-profit helping families spend generous amounts of time together.

www.familyandhome.org

International Association of Infant Massage (IAIM)

An excellent resource on baby massage.

www.iaim.net

International Lactation Consultant Association (ILCA)

World health transformed through breastfeeding and skilled lactation care.

www.ilca.org

La Leche League International

Helping moms worldwide to breastfeed through mother-to-mother encouragement, information, and education.

www.lalecheleague.org

Postpartum Support International

To speak to a volunteer about how you're feeling:

800-944-4PPD

www.postpartum.net

Magazines

Mothering

A magazine for natural family living.

www.mothering.com

New Beginnings

Published by La Leche League International

www.lalecheleague.org

Welcome Home

Published by Family and Home Network

www.familyandhome.org

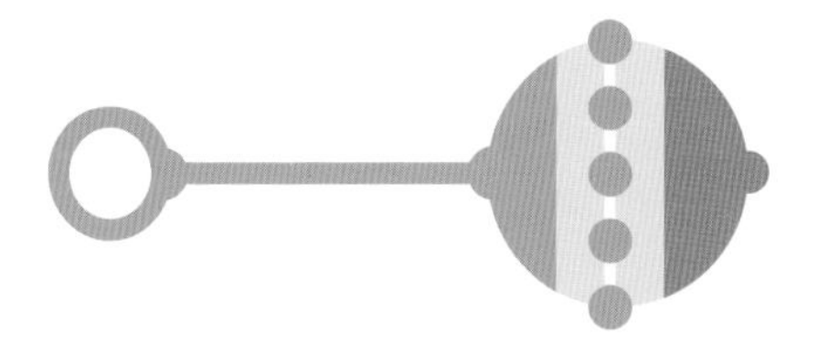

Books

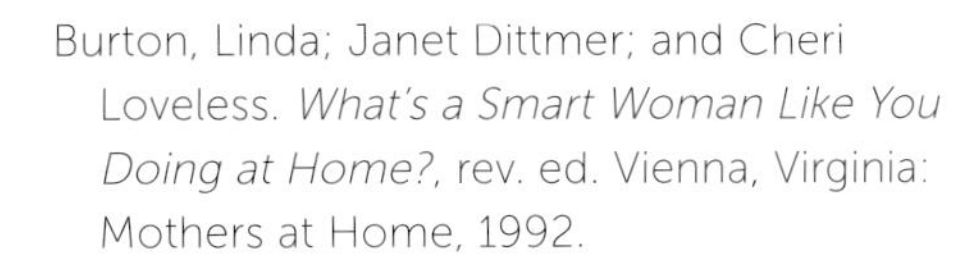

Burton, Linda; Janet Dittmer; and Cheri Loveless. *What's a Smart Woman Like You Doing at Home?*, rev. ed. Vienna, Virginia: Mothers at Home, 1992.

Gotsch, Gwen. *Breastfeeding Pure and Simple*, rev. ed. Schaumburg, Illinois: La Leche League International, 2000.

Kippley, Sheila. *Breastfeeding and Natural Child Spacing: How "Ecological" Breastfeeding Spaces Babies*, 2nd rev. ed. Cincinnati, Ohio: The Couple to Couple League, 1999. (Write the Couple to Couple League at P.O. Box 111184, Cincinnati, Ohio 45211, www.ccli.org.)

Klaus, Marshall, and Phyllis Klaus. Your *Amazing Newborn*. New York: Da Capo Press, 2000.

La Leche League International. *The Womanly Art of Breastfeeding*, 8th rev. ed. Schaumburg, Illinois: La Leche League International, 2010.

McClure, Vimala Schneider. *Infant Massage: A Handbook for Loving Parents*, rev. ed. New York: Bantam, 2000.

Sears, William, and Martha Sears. *The Attachment Parenting Book: A Commonsense Guide to Understanding and Nurturing Your Baby*. New York: Little, Brown and Company, 2001.

Sears, William, and Martha Sears. *The Baby Book: Everything You Need to Know about Your Baby from Birth to Age Two*, rev. ed. New York: Little, Brown and Company, 2013.

Sears, William, and Martha Sears. *The Breastfeeding Book: Everything You Need to Know about Nursing Your Child from Birth Through Weaning*. New York: Little, Brown and Company, 2000.

Sears, William. *The Fussy Baby Book: Parenting Your High-Need Child from Birth Through Age Five*. New York: Little, Brown and Company, 1996.

Todd, Linda. *You and Your Newborn Baby: A Guide to the First Months after Birth*. Boston: The Harvard Common Press, 1993.

Breast Pump Product Information

Contact the following companies for information about buying or renting a high-quality breast pump. Breast pumps are also available from La Leche League International and many online distributors.

Ameda
877-992-6332
www.ameda.com

Bailey Medical Engineering
800-413-3216
www.baileymed.com

Medela
800-435-8316
www.medela.com

The "Caveman" Diet

This diet, devised by William G. Crook, M.D. (*Detecting Your Hidden Allergies*, Jackson, TN: Professional Books, 1987) eliminates all common allergenic foods. You eat nothing else for two weeks but range-fed turkey and lamb, brown or white rice, baked potatoes (with salt and pepper only), one non-gassy vegetable, such as zucchini, and a non-citrus fruit, such as pear. For breakfast, you can use a rice-based beverage (available at health-food stores) with rice cereal. You also take a calcium supplement.

At the end of two weeks, you gradually add other foods to your diet, one every four days, starting with those less commonly allergenic. You avoid for the longest time dairy products, soy products, peanuts, shellfish, coffee and other foods containing caffeine, chocolate, gas-producing vegetables, tomatoes, and citrus fruits. This enables you to determine which foods in your diet are causing problems for your breastfeeding baby. Keeping a record of the foods you eat can help you correlate fussy spells with what you've eaten in the past day or so.

About the Authors

MARTHA SEARS, R.N., mother of eight children with Dr. William Sears, is a registered nurse, a former childbirth educator, a La Leche League leader, and a lactation consultant. Martha is the co-author of twenty-five parenting books and is a popular lecturer and media guest, drawing on her eighteen years of breastfeeding experience with her eight children (including Stephen, with Down Syndrome, and Lauren, her adopted daughter). Martha speaks frequently at national parenting conferences and is noted for her advice on how to handle the most common problems facing today's mothers with their changing lifestyles.

WILLIAM SEARS, one of the country's leading pediatricians, is the creator of the popular Ask Dr. Sears website. He and Martha Sears are the best-selling authors of The Sears Parenting Library.

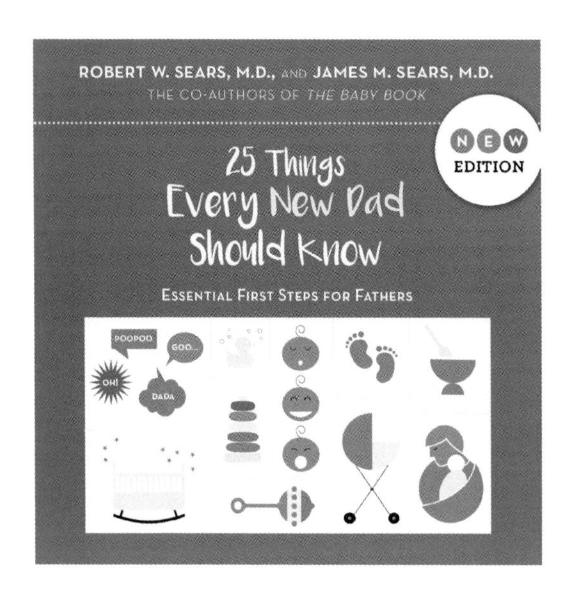

Also Available

25 Things
Every New Dad
Should Know

978-1-58832-893-8